"Jayney Goddard is ....

Natural Health

"Jayney Goddard is one of the world's leading natural health authorities. She is a true inspiration and a caring, compassionate healer."

CAMEXPO, the UK's leading professional complementary and natural healthcare annual event

"This is a truly enlightened, practical guide to taking charge of your health and longevity. Your future is in your hands – and in this book!"

Dr Mark Atkinson, MBBS, Integrative Medicine doctor and founder of the Human Potential Institute

"This book is a brilliant presentation of safe, effective and evidence-based strategies for longevity and age reversal ... Jayney Goddard's holistic vision is a rare combination of practical and scientific tools for improving function, performance, and inner and outer beauty at any age."

Frank Sabatino, DC, PhD, longevity research specialist and past Brookdale Fellow in Gerontology and Ageing

"A wonderful book by a green goddess. During my own continuing journey of trying to understand ageing and its reversal, it's become clear that you must combine science with spirituality. In this fabulous book, Jayney does just that in a clear, 'up-to-date' way. If you are into rewinding your body clock and becoming happier and healthier then you MUST read this book."

Jo Wood, former model, organic beauty brand founder and author

"Jayney's strand in our magazine has become the longest running one in our 12-year history thanks to her amazing input."

Men's Health

"Calling upon decades of experience as a leader in natural health and lifestyle medicine, Jayney provides the tools in this excellent book to help you create the healthiest, most energetic, most youthful version of yourself."

Robert Cheeke, founder and president of Vegan Bodybuilding & Fitness, author and plant-based athlete for more than 20 years

REWIND YOUR BODY CLOCK

The Complete Natural Guide
to a Happier, Healthier, Younger You

Jayney Goddard

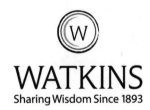

WATKINS

Sharing Wisdom Since 1893

This edition published in the UK and USA 2019 by
Watkins, an imprint of Watkins Media Limited
Unit 11, Shepperton House,
83–93 Shepperton Road,
London N1 3DF

enquiries@watkinspublishing.com

Design and typograph
Text copy

Jayney Goddard has ass
and Patents Act 1988

No part of this book r
or by any m
without prior pern

1 3 5 7 9 10 8 6 4 2

Typeset by Steve Williamson
Printed and bound in the United Kingdom

A CIP record for this book is available from the British Library

ISBN: 978-1-786782-16-8

www.watkinspublishing.com

Publisher's note: The information in this book is not intended as a substitute for professional medical advice and treatment. If you are pregnant or are suffering from any medical conditions or health problems, it is recommended that you consult a medical professional before following any of the advice or practice suggested in this book. Watkins Media Limited, or any other persons who have been involved in working on this publication, cannot accept responsibility for any injuries or damage incurred as a result of following the information, exercises or therapeutic techniques contained in this book.

ACKNOWLEDGEMENTS

In a departure from tradition, I want to start by acknowledging you, my reader. It is my sincere hope that you'll find the approaches in this book useful – both personally and for your loved ones too. I'd love to think that there is enough information in this book to help you to make sustainable, healthy, youth-enhancing changes and that you'll notice the benefits of these very quickly. I then hope, as a result, that you'll go out to become a beacon of hope and a shining example of how easy and enjoyable it is to make simple, healthy changes that really work to rewind your body clock and make you happier, healthier and younger – and in doing so that you support and encourage others to make these changes too.

What we need is a grass-roots initiative to combat the largely avoidable, and even reversible, diseases that we associate with ageing poorly. We are getting no discernible help from our governments to make these changes, so we have to take matters into our own hands. Please get out and spread the word and become one of the grass-roots team that will be the generation that truly makes a difference to the health, vitality and wellbeing of your nation.

I'd next like to express my deepest gratitude to all at Watkins for their trust in me and this book – and, in particular, Kelly Thompson, who just "has the eye". She "got" this book right from our first meeting and has, ever since, been its biggest champion. Georgie in Watkins' design department took my crazy ideas for a cover concept and magically created a beautiful artwork for it and more. I must thank my eagle-eyed editor, the brilliantly creative Sandy Draper, who did an astounding job refining this text. A huge thanks also to Vikki Scott, my talented, and frankly brilliant, publicist who has worked so hard to ensure that the important and potentially life-saving overall message of this book gets out to a vast audience, worldwide. My agent, Valeria Huerta, got the ball rolling in the first place and found my absolute dream publishers, and she also introduced me to Karen Hockney, who was invaluable in the early days in refining my initial pitch to the publishers.

My family has been an inspiration for this book, and my mother, Jill Lucas, in particular is one of the main reasons that I rebelled against the medical status quo and chose the more natural path that I now find myself on. In the 1970s, she experienced a very long, extremely debilitating illness, which was, unforgivably, misdiagnosed several times – medical misogyny being even more prevalent back then. Eventually, she was diagnosed with type 1 diabetes.

Now, back in the 1970s, diabetics had to follow a very rigid regime of specified insulin doses and she had to weigh every morsel of food to calculate its carbohydrate content. Mum, being the brilliant woman that she is – and always a rebel – soon realized that this accepted system wasn't natural, or even remotely reflective of "real life". So, she started to adjust her insulin intake to account for the food that she'd eaten and the amount of activity that she'd done. She felt that she was mimicking the action of a normally functioning pancreas. This seemed very logical to her and she was doing brilliantly; her blood sugar levels were perfect, with very few spikes or troughs. However, when she told her doctors what she was doing, their response was "You're crazy, you're going to die!" But Mum, being Mum, just carried on – and continued to get wonderful blood sugar readings and felt better than she had done in years.

In the end, an enlightened consultant looked at her approach and decided that she was really on to something pretty special, so he ran a trial and discovered that Mum's approach was, in fact, ideal! It now has a name – DAFNE (Dose Adjustment For Normal Eating) – and Jill was the inspiration for this. So, I learned at a very early age that you can't rely upon the status quo and that sometimes it pays to rebel and find a new and better way. And that's what we are doing in this book.

I want to thank Dr Frank Sabatino, DC, PhD, for his brilliance, kindness, endless encouragement and advice. It's a funny story, because in all my years of research and writing about the scientific side of biological age reversal, I found myself repeatedly referencing published research papers by "Sabatino, F.D.", one of the leading scientists in the gerontology field. Now, as luck would have it, I was introduced to a charming American doctor by our mutual friend Bethany Vinal, and, a few months later, the penny dropped and I realized that this lovely man was, in fact, the "Sabatino, F.D." that I'd been referencing and inspired by, all these years.

Finally, I say a huge thank you to Roberta MacMillan (aka Wonder Woman), vice president of The CMA, who keeps everything running smoothly even when I'm deeply engrossed in writing. To Bianca and Patrizia – always great sounding boards and loyal friends. To Lesley Lucas, kindness and wisdom personified. And last, but by no means least, to my dear friends, an eclectic bunch of wise women, dancers, scientists, artists and more who may be scattered far wide but who live together, always, in my heart.

"This book is dedicated to all you trail-blazing 'Rewind Rebels' who know that our health, happiness and vibrant, youthful longevity is in our own hands – and that the wise choices we make today will safeguard not just our own wellbeing, but also that of our planet!"

CONTENTS

HAPPIER AND HEALTHIER FROM THE INSIDE OUT

If you are looking for a way to stay young, healthy, vibrant, smart and sexy, you're in the right place! We all know that there are an abundance of synthetic and cosmetic quick fixes out there that can make a real difference to our appearance right away. These can be effective, and certainly have their place, but if, like me, you want to create a truly effervescent life that just fizzes with energy and joy, you'll need to harness the amazingly effective, easy-to-follow tips in this book.

The recommendations in this book aren't just skin deep, but can quite literally reverse your biological age. Admittedly, the term "biological age" is a bit of a dry one, and I don't think anyone has ever said, "I want to be biologically younger!" But given the hundreds of billions spent on anti-ageing products and services, it's a fairly safe bet to assume that most of us do want to age well, and feel and look as youthful as possible. So, you'll find the term "biological ageing" popping up a lot in this book. It takes into consideration the functioning of your body, your chemistry and physiology, your cognitive performance, your mental acuity and more. It differs from your chronological age, which is simply a measurement of your age in years. It is quite possible for your biological age to be very different from your chronological age, as you'll learn in this book.

An Evidence-Based Approach

I'll be your guide on this exciting adventure and I feel that it's important to tell you that all the approaches in this book are backed by proper scientific research. So, while we are using natural, holistic techniques, this is not some pie-in-the-sky manifesto of wishful thinking. On the contrary, while my approaches are fun and fulfilling (and sometimes perhaps a little off the wall), everything you will read here actually works. In short, this is your most direct and rapid route to long-lasting health and outstanding wellbeing: mentally, emotionally, physically and spiritually. If we are healthy in all these areas of ourselves then we will look, feel and function better in every way.

Mindset and Lifestyle Choices for Optimal Health

One of the most overlooked facts in our culture is that many of the chronic diseases that we associate with ageing are avoidable, and even reversible – and most of them are related to our mindset and lifestyle choices. The problem that we, as a society, face is that these diseases not only take a terrible toll on the individual and their loved ones, but on society too, as they are incredibly expensive conditions to treat. But all the research shows that if we know how to look after ourselves, cook wholefoods from scratch, exercise well and manage our stress response, the picture would be very different.

So, this is why I felt it necessary to write this book: it is my hope that you'll be inspired to make enjoyable, healthy changes for yourself and your loved ones and that you'll also be able to help get the message out there on a wider level; that good health is our birthright, and that very simple steps can make a huge difference to us all – and to society. We have to act now, or it really will be too late.

Throughout the book you'll find a lot of references to scientific studies and research programmes, which make for fascinating reading, so if you're interested in diving deeper into any of this evidence then head on over to my website, JayneyGoddard.org, for a full list of references.

Why Me?

As we're going to be companions on this journey, you might like to know a little more about me. Needless to say, I'm passionate about social change in healthcare – it's why I trained as a complementary medical practitioner over 30 years ago.

I spent my first seven years training in homeopathy and Ericksonian Analysis and have since trained in a range of additional natural healthcare disciplines including Reiki, lifestyle medicine, medical qigong and more. I'm deeply dedicated to being the best practitioner I can be so that I can offer the most appropriate and effective therapeutic options to my patients. In 2012, I trained in Mind/Body Medicine at Harvard Medical School, under Dr Herbert Benson, considered to be the "Father" of Mind/Body Medicine. Before that, I graduated from the University of Central Lancashire with an MSc, as I have always been committed to ensuring that there is a strong scientific basis for all my recommendations.

I've been in practice for the past 25 years, but my work also necessitates huge amounts of international travel, crossing time zones and often burning the candle at both ends. This is a challenge for anyone, even if they're in the best of health, but, despite the hand of cards I was dealt from my genetic deck – I suffer from rheumatoid arthritis – I have managed to elevate my health and wellbeing using the approaches in this book so that I can sustain the energy levels needed to maintain an incredibly busy, energetic (and happy) life.

My Story

I first became fascinated by biological age reversal and effectively rewound my own body clock 17 years ago. It's a strange story. Although I had been really struggling with the rheumatoid arthritis – and had been a full-time wheelchair user for ten years – things didn't really become "life or death" until I experienced an enormous flare-up in 2001.

At that point, I was admitted into a hospice and told that I had two weeks to "get my affairs in order", as I really wasn't expected to live. Due to the excruciating pain, I was completely immobile – locked into a foetal position. With rheumatoid arthritis, many people assume that just the joints that are affected, but it is an autoimmune disease, which means that your body attacks itself in its entirety – so it can be a life-threatening condition. So, during this devastating flare-up, not only were my joints dangerously inflamed, as you might expect, but so were my internal organs, including my brain, liver, kidneys, lungs and blood vessels. My whole system was under attack and it was quite terrifying.

Before my admission into the hospice, I was eating everything in sight to try to maintain my weight – but each day it dropped another 2lbs. I was stuffing the highest-calorie food into my body that I could lay my hands on, every single night. I'd eat a large pizza with all the toppings and extra cheese, followed by a tub of ice cream, and then perhaps another tub of ice cream. And, yet, my weight was still plummeting – until I reached 77lbs (34.9kg; 5.5 stone). (As you'll read later in the book, I was doing everything wrong. In my struggle to save my life, I was driving the inflammation that was killing me – little did I know.)

Despite the medics' dire prognosis, I knew enough to realize that there must be something that could be done to calm down the runaway inflammation. In an effort to find a solution, I was trying lots of different approaches and tests in order to figure out what would be the best for me. One of the tests that provided an indication of biological age came back with a reading of 55 years old, which was pretty tough to hear as I was only 36 at the time!

I therefore started to throw everything I had at my health problem – all my training, as well as treatments and advice from my trusted health practitioner colleagues. And, little by little, I figured out what I needed to do. When it became apparent that I was going to survive, I was discharged from the hospice and moved to a high-dependency residential unit. I stayed there for nearly a year – still working on myself. And, slowly, I returned to health by developing and following my own unique and holistic mind/body approach to reach deep, lasting, vibrant wellness. This is the same approach that I continue to follow today and recommend to my patients. I know that the mind/body practices I recommend work because, after I recovered, I made a point of regularly testing my biological age. So, I retested a year after my health meltdown, and I discovered that my biological age had reverted to 27. Amazing! However, what's even more interesting is that 17 years later, at the age of 55, I'm still measuring at 27 biologically – so not only have my approaches rewound my body clock, they have also profoundly slowed my biological age progression.

Now, I appreciate that my story alone is not proof that any of my methods will work for you, but you might be interested to hear that many of my patients have experienced similarly dramatic reversals in age biomarkers. Furthermore, biological age reversal – or, in more poetic terms, "the search for the fountain of youth" – is something that scientists have been researching for quite some time. Age reversal and the prevention of the diseases we associate with ageing is one of the hottest topics in science today and there have been numerous trials that amply demonstrate the effectiveness of all the elements in my approach.

My Passion for Health

Over the years, I have built an international following, and I have to credit that to the fact that everything I teach is easy and enjoyable to implement, and that my patients see real changes – fast. Even some of the trickiest health problems can be helped to some degree by making lifestyle changes – and of course as soon as people notice real change, they are telling friends and family to come along to see me too. To me, this is proof that what I'm doing is really making a difference in people's lives.

Alongside my practice, I realized that there needed to be a standardization across the board in complementary and integrative medicine as a whole to ensure that practitioners offered the very best to their patients – both in terms of safety and effectiveness. Back in 1993, after I had first graduated, there was nothing available in terms of a society that could realistically bring together practitioners and training schools of all disciplines, and so I founded The Complementary Medical Association (The CMA), which has, over the years, become the world's largest and most respected professional membership association in natural healthcare.

We are a global organization and I work closely with governments across the world to help them standardize complementary medicine – so that patients and doctors know exactly who is properly qualified and can offer the very best treatments. I was even tasked by the USA's White House Commission on Complementary and Alternative Medicine Policy to look at all forms of natural healthcare across all 50 states and to standardize them. As you can imagine, it was a huge task – but also hugely gratifying, as all my recommendations were accepted unanimously.

I've had some other real adventures along the way too. For example, I did a similar task for the Bulgarian and Hungarian governments – who have a fantastic history of balneotherapy (water cure), where patients are treated in the most amazing medical spas. They bathe in and drink the mineral waters there and, alongside that, lots of other treatments are on offer, including their shocking electrical bath (yes, an actual bath with an electrical current running through it – imagine an all-over TENS machine) and the water traction device (you are suspended by your head in deep water and left hanging, literally. Great for sorting out any spinal kinks and provoking deep relaxation, believe it or not). And, yes, in the spirit of science, I tried them all.

Achievements Worth Noting

I'm now going to brag a little – just a little – so please bear with me. I promise it's for a good reason. I believe that when you embark on a truly life-changing adventure – and this book is just that – you need to know that your guide actually has some credibility and might know a thing or two about the topic. So, here goes …

Bringing complementary medicine to a truly professional footing globally means I have received many awards and accolades along the way.

These include:

- Winning the CAMEXPO Award for Outstanding Contribution to Complementary Medicine
- Being named Honorary International Advisor and awarded a Professorship by the Kingdom of Nepal
- Founding the USA's Integrative Healthcare Symposium
- Being an Honorary Advisor to the Health Food Manufacturers' Association
- Founding and co-chairing the British Society for Lifestyle Medicine
- Being president of The Complementary Medical Association

I also hold Fellowships of both the Royal Society of Medicine and the Royal Society for Public Health. So, nowadays, when I'm not seeing my patients and running The CMA, I'm writing, broadcasting and speaking all over the world – often at medical schools (including recently at the University of Cambridge and the University of Miami Miller School of Medicine), where the students, and the faculty more often than not, want to learn about what really works in complementary medicine – and where to go for the actual proof. I'm also incredibly fortunate to be the columnist for *Natural Health* magazine and to act as the natural healthcare expert for Discovery Health, as well as writing for various national newspapers.

Where It All Began

Of course, I didn't set out to be an expert on anti-ageing, but the calling happened many years ago, when I was a teenager, training to be a ballet dancer. My goal at that time was to get an Equity Contract (similar to the Screen Actors Guild in the USA). So, there were auditions at my ballet school and a coveted Equity Contract was proffered, and it turned out that the job was actually working as a dancer in a circus. But this was no ordinary circus; it was a static Big Top in Battersea Park, London, featuring the very best circus acts from around the world. I remember meeting and greeting Princess Margaret, Mick Jagger and Jerry Hall – and, in a tricky guest list twist, Brian Ferry and his then-partner. I also remember meeting heart-throb David Essex, most of the Osmonds and more. It was a real head-turner for a 16-year-old. To cut a long story short, quite naturally, I fell madly in love with the dashing Colombian high-wire walker and decided that going back to ballet school was way too boring a prospect, so, in a truly clichéd move, I ran away with the circus. Now, obviously, I wasn't on a free ride. I had to earn my keep, so I learnt how to do aerial and trapeze work. When you are a teenager, you have no concept of your own mortality and the thought of falling never even occurred to me. Nevertheless, we did have a few relatively minor accidents, and we were travelling in some pretty remote places all over the world. There were always sprains and cuts, and in my case "elephant hair chaffing", as I doubled up as an elephant rider/acrobat, and elephants have very stiff and pointy, scratchy hairs. (In circuses, you often have to double up and do various acts – so yes, in the spirit of full disclosure, I was also a magician's assistant and have been shot out of a cannon!)

In most of the places we worked, there was no access to conventional medicine, so in the case of injury, the local shaman, witch doctor or wise woman was summoned and we were treated with herbs, potions and all manner of concoctions. And we got better – fast! Despite being in some very primitive environments, often without running water or electricity, no one ever contracted an infection. I found this remarkable. And when, after four years as a circus artiste, I went back to the UK, dancing in West End shows and the like, I couldn't shift this fascination with the incredibly powerful, effective jungle medicines I'd seen. It got to the point that I was so entranced that I decided that the way forward was to study homeopathic medicine, and it was one of the best things I have ever done, as it catapulted me – much like a lady being shot out of a cannon! – right into the complementary medical field, and I haven't looked back since!

An Inside Job

As you'll appreciate, I'm now doing everything I can to get the message out that we are so much more in control of our own health – and how we age – than we can even begin to realize. And, given that humans are incredibly complex individuals, it won't surprise you to hear that our mindset is as important as our lifestyle if we want to hold on to our youth.

Staying youthful is of huge importance to so many people, myself included, and I have many friends who will do pretty much anything to hold on to their vitality, attractiveness, intelligence, physical fitness and mental acuity. Just take a look at any beauty counter or glossy magazine and you'll see products and articles all promising to reverse the signs of ageing. The pursuit of youthful vitality is so important to us as a society that the size of the anti-ageing industry was estimated at over $250 billion in 2016 and estimated to reach $331.41 billion by 2020. It is a field that is developing so fast that no true figure can be placed on the size of the market; it is akin to an avalanche.

Vast sums are spent by people desperate for the quick fix, which can be disastrous; we are all familiar with the stars who have had botched plastic surgeries. And yet there are others who know when to stop and look "well" rather than "done". I believe that the difference between these two sets of people is that those who sadly get botched don't have a long-term commitment to health and internal wellbeing, whereas the other set of people – like Jane Fonda for instance – have had a lifelong commitment to health and wellbeing, and this enables them to heal better from any surgery. And, of course, they have the kind of mindset that enables them to know what to do – and, more importantly, when to stop.

While many people tend to think of vanity as something superfluous, narcissistic or egotistical, it isn't always so. In fact, a healthy dose of vanity is intrinsically important to our mental, physical and physiological wellbeing and, by default, maintenance of a younger biological age. Taking pride in your appearance is, in itself, a marker of youthfulness. Conversely, one indication of the start of a descent into premature decline and an unhealthy old age is someone giving up and no longer making any effort to present themselves well, both privately and in public. Vanity is a little bit "chicken and egg": when we take pride in our appearance, we feel better, and vice versa.

Intriguingly, this is just one of the clues that will help us to decode the ageing conundrum. Ageing is not linear and is not subject to simple cause and effect. It is much more complex than this, and it may be that our mindset has more impact on ageing than we could ever imagine.

Ageing: Is It All in the Mind?

It is entirely possible that up to 95 per cent or more of our mindset and beliefs about ageing actually influence how well we age. It is such a vital part of the ageing puzzle, yet it is often overlooked, which is why I decided to make it an important component of this book. Of course, nutrition, exercise, etc. are all hugely important, but if our mindset isn't right, then everything else we do risks being a waste of time.

It's impossible to overestimate the importance of the way we relate to society's subliminal messages about how we are supposed to be at any particular point in our lives; unfortunately, our culture fosters expectations of an inevitable decline into illness and infirmity.

Ellen Langer, PhD, a professor of psychology from Harvard Medical School, has turned this erroneous notion on its head by carrying out research that has shown how, given the right circumstances, we can reverse our age, not chronologically of course, but biologically. In fact, Langer believes that we have almost complete mental control over our diseases, including the conditions we perceive to be an inevitable counterpart to ageing (for more information, go to EllenLanger.com).

One of the most influential and intriguing studies by Langer is the Counter Clockwise study first carried out in 1979 (and replicated for a BBC documentary called *The Young Ones* in 2010 with even more astonishing results). Two groups of men were divided into a control group and an experimental group. The control group attended a retreat where they spent a week reminiscing about the past. Meanwhile, the experimental group spent a week in an environment where all surrounding sensory clues, such as decor, music and food, pointed to a time when the men were 20 years younger and felt at their best, to see if this would make them feel and *act* as if they were younger. By the end of the study, this group demonstrated marked improvement in benchmark health tests such as hearing, eyesight, memory, dexterity and appetite, while there was no change in the control group.

And if more proof were needed about the effect of our minds and perceptions on our ageing process, Professor Langer has also demonstrated a strong link between a certain type of male-pattern baldness and an increase in the risk of prostate cancer. Prostate cancer is more common in older men, and Langer and her colleagues believe that this might be because balding men feel older every time they look in a mirror and get a visual reminder that they appear to be ageing. In addition, some heart problems are also linked to balding, despite there being no obvious biological rationale for a connection between the two, hence the

Rewind Insight: "Lifespan" and "health-span" are two important terms that you will encounter in this book. My hope is that they will help you to cultivate a mindset shift that will allow you to view health and wellbeing from a different, more empowered, perspective. We are all aware that the term "lifespan" means the number of years that we live – but "health-span" is a much more important and relevant term as it indicates the number of years we live healthily and free of disease. So, sadly, in industrialized nations, while our lifespan is generally increasing, our health-span is decreasing. This book sets out to change all that!

researchers hypothesizing that the men's mindsets about their age could be partly responsible.

So, if Ellen Langer and her colleagues are right that feeling, looking and behaving more youthfully ultimately makes you healthier, what should we do? She is quite clear when she says, "Don't buy the mindset in the first place. Then you won't be vulnerable to it. I think we have far more control over our health and wellbeing than most of us realize."

Consciously Choosing Your Mindset

If we aren't going to buy into the myths that society tries to sell us about ageing, it follows that we have to work on developing a more positive mindset for ourselves in terms of how we view ageing, right?

In this book, I therefore take a deep dive into steps that you can take to ensure that you develop the youthful, vibrant outlook that really will help you to rewind your body clock.

See the exercise opposite for a helpful – and fun! – exercise that, as silly as it may sound, really does have the power to enhance your frame of mind by making you feel younger, more vibrant and more free.

In addition, I have included a positive mindset phrase at the start of each chapter of Part II, to ensure that you get into a proactive frame of mind from the outset with each topic. And I've also added a prompt to come up with your own positive and specific Mindset Phrase at the end of each of these chapters (see more on how to get the most from these features overleaf, on page 13).

Let's Get This Show on the Road

It's my hope that the information in this book will guide you on an exciting adventure toward both looking and feeling more youthful – with more energy, greater happiness, more resilience against stress, improved hormonal balance, better brain and cognitive function, enhanced libido and much more. Please do also go to my website (JayneyGoddard.org) to access further material to support your age reversal. Rest assured that we're in this together, and I can't wait to begin the journey with you!

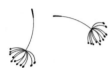

REWIND ANCHOR PRACTICE
Mindset Immersion Therapy

Any time you're feeling tired or old, take inspiration from Professor Langer's groundbreaking research (see page 9) by surrounding yourself with "youth cues" to remind yourself, whether consciously or subconsciously, of when you were biologically at your prime. For most of us, this would be when we were in the midst of a powerful growth spurt in our mid-teens, or maybe in our twenties. The following Rewind suggestions are my adaptation of Professor Langer's "immersion" experiment. My clients swear by it, and so do I. Have fun!

- Put on music you adored when you were a teenager and sing along as loud as you want and/or dance around the living room to it.
- Track down some back copies of whatever magazines you read at the time and set aside a little time to leaf through them at leisure.
- Spend time looking back at your pin-ups and idols of that era. Try not to laugh. Remember: this is doing you good!
- Look back over old photos to trigger fond memories and friendships from this period.
- Create time for activities that you loved doing then and that you were good at, whether that be dancing, acting, playing hockey, doing craft activities or whatever else.
- Invite friends of a similar age to a "Rewind Party" where you play music you all loved and maybe even choose retro nibbles and drinks. Think of it as an old-school disco.
- Try and dress the part. Honestly, it really will help. It's time to get a dressing-up box if you don't already have one!
- Reminisce about who you fancied then, the bands you loved and the fashions and hairstyles you wore (no matter how much they might make you cringe now!)
- Lastly, do let your friends in on why you are doing this – you don't want them thinking you have lost the plot! And, of course, if they join in, they too will reap the anti-ageing benefits of your wild, yet powerfully effective and fun experiment.

GETTING THE MOST FROM YOUR REWIND JOURNEY

Given that you are reading this book, I think it is safe to assume that you have a strong desire to rewind your body clock. Obviously, there are different motivations for each of us, so it's important to explore which is most relevant to you. Here are some common reasons that I encounter when I'm with my patients:

- I'm interested in preserving my health so that I can live longer more healthily.
- I want to look and feel better, younger, sexier, brainer.
- I need to stay in the workplace for longer/I love my work and don't want to retire early (or at all).
- I just want to have more fun in my life and I recognize the importance of maintaining vibrant, youthful health in facilitating this.
- I'm concerned that I might inherit the same condition as my parents or grandparents – and I want to avoid this.
- I just want to look good naked. (*Don't we all?*)
- I love life and want to stay healthy, happy and more energetic and youthful for longer.

Do any of these apply to you? Or is there anything missing that speaks to you more directly? If so, note your thoughts down to help inspire you. These notes will also be something that you can come back to to see how you're faring as you work through the tips and techniques in the book. Below is a list of more specific benefits of reading this book, which may help you to hone your ideas on this front:

- Feel more energetic – no more afternoon slumps.
- Get more youthful-looking skin – any fine lines and wrinkles will lessen, you'll heal faster from cuts and bruises, and hormonal-based breakouts will disappear.
- Help your hair grow thicker and faster with effective home remedies.
- Enhance your thinking processes and memory.
- Develop stress resilience: stress is inevitable, but it is how you *respond* to stressors that dictates how much of a toll they will take on your health – and biological age. The more susceptible you are to stress, the "older" you will be in biological terms.
- Use simple meditation exercises to "rewire" your brain so that you become less "reactive" – which is a huge benefit when faced with stress
- Use easy, enjoyable practices to make you feel happier overall and dramatically increase your compassion levels – for yourself and others.
- Draw from the mighty power of medicinal herbs for wellness, to boost your libido and balance your hormones.
- Explore strategies for incorporating nature into your daily life, because a deep connection to nature is extremely youth-promoting.
- Enjoy more healing, revitalizing sleep.

The Book Structure

In order to make the information in the book both as practical and easy to use as possible, I have chosen to present it in three distinct sections:

- **Part I – Your Rewind Mindset:**
  Understanding Ageing and Reframing How You View It

- **Part II – Your Rewind Toolkit:**
  Empowering Yourself to Turn Back the Years

- **Part III – Your 21-Day Rewind Plan:**
  Taking Immediate Action

Part I – Your Rewind Mindset

This initial section lays the foundations for the rest of the book by exploring the key concepts related to ageing, such as the science behind the ageing process, the effect that our genetic make-up can have on us, what we can do to keep the damaging powers of inflammation at bay and how much more power we have over our mind and body than we often realize. Dotted throughout the book you will find occasional "Rewind Insight" features that give you handy extra explanations, tips and techniques. You will also find exercises in this section called "Rewind Anchor Practices". These will help set you up for your Rewind Journey. They can also be done at any other time that you feel you need a boost during your journey toward both feeling and looking younger.

While it's not essential that you read *all* of this section if it doesn't appeal to you, doing so will give you a strong context from which to understand all the information then presented in the rest of the book.

Part II – Your Rewind Toolkit

This second section of the book is where you will find all the practical information you need to take a holistic, multifunctional approach to slowing down and/or reversing your ageing process. As such, you'll find that there are chapters on nutrition, gut health, supplements, fasting, herbs, breathwork, exercise, skin care, hair care, hormonal balance, relationships, nature and sleep – all of which have an impact on how well you age. It's entirely up to you whether you choose to read each chapter systematically, topic by topic, or if you'd prefer to start by dipping into the chapters that seem most immediately relevant to you. In the end, however, it certainly would prove useful to read all the chapters when you have time, given that a sense of holistic balance is so key to both looking and feeling young and vibrant for as long as possible. In each chapter within this section, you will find:

- A positive Mindset Phrase at the start to help get you into the most receptive state of mind for the content to come. I recommend that you repeat this to yourself several times, whether out loud or in your own head, before you read the rest of the chapter.
- Practical exercises and tips entitled "Rewind Practice: Over to You" for you to experiment with and find the approaches that best suit you. I firmly believe that if you have techniques that you enjoy, you are far more likely to stick to them – and in biological age reversal, it's "stickability" that counts!
- A prompt at the end of each chapter where I encourage you to come up with your own, more specific and personal positive Mindset Phrase related to the theme in hand, to help you clarify in your own mind exactly how you are going to use the information in your everyday life! See overleaf for some guidance on how best to formulate these in order to maximize the benefits you gain from each chapter.

Here are a few useful rules to follow when coming up with your own Mindset Phrase at the end of each chapter:

- Make the content as positive and proactive as possible.
- Keep a note of each one somewhere central, such as in a journal or online in your secure log-in section at JayneyGoddard.org, so that you have them all together as a reference for assessment in the future.
- Write them in the present tense (rather than the future tense) so that your subconscious mind starts to act as if the content is already real. This will make the actions much easier to turn into reality as your mind will be unable to separate thoughts from reality.
- Make them as specific as possible. So, for example, instead of saying something like "I am improving my diet" or "I am constantly improving my health by making nurturing food choices", it is more effective to say something like "I am improving my life by choosing to eat delicious salads with a rainbow of veggies as often as possible". And instead of saying "I work out every day", it would be better to say something like "I lift weights and do my resistance exercises every other day, alternating with yoga on other days". This way you give your mind really *specific* guidance in terms of what to do. And the more specific you can be, the more likely you will be to reap the rewards.

Writing these Mindset Phrases may feel a bit weird at first, as if you are "making things up" – and perhaps you are at the beginning – but it really doesn't matter because your brain will accept the statements as truths, which will help you in your quest to feel more youthful and vibrant.

Part III – Your 21-Day Rewind Plan

This is where you'll find a specially designed programme, presented on a day-by-day basis over three full weeks, to help you start integrating all the recommendations in the book into your daily life. You'll also find out here how to access all my special, reader-only downloads and online tracking tools, so that you can measure just how well you are doing.

Do feel free to let me know at any point how you're getting on by joining my private "Rewind Your Body Clock" Facebook group, which I have set up as a way to support you in your journey and also as a place for us all to interact and learn from each other. When you are making any lifestyle changes, it really helps to be surrounded by like-minded people who are on the same adventure as you. All the research shows that peer support definitely improves results – no matter what your goals are!

REWIND ANCHOR PRACTICE
Setting Your Motivations and Goals

Getting clarity on your motivations and goals will be key to you getting the most from this book, so below is a chart for you to use as inspiration to create a list of both things that you would like more of in your life and things that you would like less of. Once you have completed these lists, it should be easier for you to decide which chapters in the book you might like to spend most time and energy on.

There's not much room in the chart below, so I'd suggest recreating it in a notebook or your journal. Alternatively, you can complete the one online at JayneyGoddard.org, as it makes it so much easier to keep everything in one place for the next time you repeat the exercise. Either way, be sure to use the present tense for each statement that you write, as per the advice just given for the Mindset Phrases that you'll encounter later in the book. For example, you might end up including statements such as "I have more energy to enjoy the things I love", "I spend more time dancing", "I get out into nature more", "I let go of self-doubt", "I eat a lot less sugar than I used to" or "I no longer suffer from frequent headeaches."

Feel free to add as many points as you like. And, once you have completed the lists, number each column of statements in priority order, with No. I being the most important thing you want to achieve.

I have/do more ...	I have/do less ...

These lists will be a useful tool for you to refer back to when it comes to creating your Mindset Phrase at the end of each chapter in Part II – to ensure that each one is aligned with your key underlying motivations and goals. They will also be a handy point of reference in terms of tracking your progress as time moves on. However, do be aware, of course, that your priorities may change as you work through the book, so feel free to come back to the lists and update them at any time.

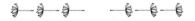

SELF-ASSESSMENT
WHERE ARE YOU NOW?

Before we go any further, your first assignment is to go through the following checklists, and subsequent simple DIY tests, to get a snapshot of where you are with your health and biological age right now.

Please don't freak out, however, if you find that you are ticking absolutely everything on the list or don't get the results you would like in the tests. I certainly found this when I was going through my own health meltdown! I have bounced back to abundant health by using all the recommendations in this book – and if I can do it, I'm certain you can too!

Getting an Overview

Feel free to copy the list before starting if you'd rather not write in the book. Then go through each point and simply tick the box beside it if the issue mentioned is one you suffer from.

In order to make it a more useful tool for you, give yourself a rating between 1 and 5 for each of the issues that you acknowledge with a tick, where 1 is the worst you feel this particular aspect of ageing could be and 5 is the best it could be. This is obviously by no means a technical way of recording things, but it will give you a good sense of how you feel about where you are each time you do the self-assessment.

You can then come back to this list and go through it again roughly every month – as a useful way of tracking your progress over time. I have also put the list up on JayneyGoddard.org.

Skin

☐ Fine lines and wrinkles, especially on the face, neck and décolleté
☐ Lack of skin suppleness: the skin on the back of your hand doesn't bounce back when pinched (see the Skin Pinch Test on page 24)

- ☐ Age spots
- ☐ Discolouration
- ☐ Cellulite

Musculoskeletal
- ☐ Muscle shrinkage: smaller muscles and wrinkled skin over muscles (e.g. at the top and on inside of the arm in women)
- ☐ Flabby triceps (bingo wings)
- ☐ Loss of strength, such as when carrying things
- ☐ Diminished grip strength
- ☐ Inability to rise from the floor hands-free
- ☐ Arthritis
- ☐ Aching joints
- ☐ Osteopenia: your bones are weaker than normal but not so far gone that they break easily, which is the hallmark of osteoporosis
- ☐ Osteoporosis: when your bones have deteriorated so much that you are at high risk of sustaining a fracture
- ☐ Bone spurs: these occur more frequently as we age
- ☐ Reduced flexibility (see the Flexibility Test on page 27–28)

Eyes
- ☐ Vision changes: becoming long-sighted or other eyesight changes. If you've made no other lifestyle changes, this can be a sign of ageing.
- ☐ Dry eyes
- ☐ Distorted or changed vision: if this is sudden and unexplained, get it checked out by a professional immediately

Ears
- ☐ Diminished hearing

Hair
- ☐ Hair loss
- ☐ Hair thinning
- ☐ Hair greying
- ☐ Loss of shine and bounce
- ☐ Poorer condition
- ☐ Frizziness/dryness

Appetite and Thirst

☐ Diminished or excessive appetite

☐ Diminished sense of taste: we can sometimes find that we need ever more sugar or salt, in order to be able to taste our food

☐ Less thirst: as we age we become less sensitive to "thirst signals", which can quickly lead to dehydration

Bowel and Urinary Tract

☐ Bowel changes (e.g. more loose stools or frequent constipation)

☐ Greater susceptibility to urinary tract infections (UTIs)

☐ More frequent urination

☐ Urinary leakage or stress incontinence (e.g. peeing from laughing, jumping or any exertion)

☐ Piles/haemorrhoids

☐ If you notice blood in your stools, or tarry-looking stools, or if you notice blood when you wipe (after having a wee), get checked out by your doctor immediately

Sex

☐ Reduced libido (if sudden, with no logical explanation): sadly, lack of sex drive in women is often "pathologized" when there is a perfectly logical explanation for it. I see this a lot in my practice, particularly in cases where a woman's male partner is no longer appealing to them.

☐ Painful intercourse (if sudden, with no logical explanation)

☐ Physical issues including vaginal atrophy, thinning vaginal skin and prolapse. Prolapse is serious and requires immediate medical attention.

Sleep

☐ Insomnia

☐ Restlessness

☐ Night sweats

Brain/Mind

☐ Poor/reduced concentration

☐ Poor/worsening short-term and/or long-term memory

☐ Reduced ability to comprehend something you've just read

General

☐ Greater susceptibility to colds/flu or other infections

☐ Difficulty regulating temperature

- ☐ Sensitive startle response (e.g. easily startled by an unexpected noise)
- ☐ Poorer balance
- ☐ Reduced reaction speed
- ☐ Poor "body composition" (e.g. you'd like more muscle and less fat)
- ☐ Menopausal symptoms (e.g. hot flushes (flashes), mood changes, etc.)
- ☐ Any of the so-called diseases of ageing:
  - ☐ type 2 diabetes
  - ☐ high blood pressure
  - ☐ arthritis (osteo)
  - ☐ heart disease
  - ☐ lifestyle-related cancers
  - ☐ neurological problems
  - ☐ any other condition/s you have at the moment that you'd like to address

Well done for completing this list. Please come back to it in a month's time, either here, on your copied-out version, or online, at JayneyGoddard.org, so that you can track your changes.

Official Testing Option

It is possible to get official blood tests to gauge your biological age by measuring your telomere length, antioxidant status and more (you'll be learning more about these topics later in the book). However, I would approach such tests with some caution. They are very pricey, and for them to be meaningful, you'd have to keep repeating them to see how well any age-reversal strategies you are putting into place are progressing.

Aside from the expense, accuracy is also a concern, because if you have your telomere length measured, it will only reflect how that particular body part or system is doing; it won't reflect on your cognitive function, your response and reflex rate, your flexibility and balance, skin elasticity and much more. Yet all these factors combined are intrinsically related to our overall biological age picture. We are, after all, human beings, and we operate as a constellation of entire systems working together. Just measuring one part alone doesn't reflect what's going on as a whole.

There are also lab-based biological age tests that use more than just telomere length as their marker, but, again, if you were even able to access equipment to do these tests privately, they would be extremely expensive.

Finally, there are lots of online questionnaires available. By all means do them, but I *personally* don't believe that they are necessarily that accurate, as they tend to fail to provide parameters within their structure that account for the huge variability in our life circumstances. Plus, many of them use contradictory parameters to measure age. I recently came across one, for example, that penalized you in terms of biological age if you drank any alcohol at all and another one that penalized you if you drank *no* alcohol. There's some logic to both approaches, but, ultimately, there's just so much conflicting information about alcohol consumption that it renders both tests void.

Home Tests

There are, however, some relatively simple and reliable tests that you can do at home. While they won't give you a definitive age – again, for the reasons explained above – they are generally used in biological age testing as their results are both trackable and meaningful. Plus, they are free to do! In the pages that follow you will find eight tests in total:

- Skin Pinch Test
- Balance Test
- Vision Test
- Ruler Drop Reaction Time Test
- Flexibility Test
- Wall Sit Test
- Waist Measurement
- Height Measurement

Some of these were used in the BBC programme *The Young Ones* that I mentioned at the beginning of the book. This fantastic programme was presented by the always excellent Dr Michael Mosley and the ultimate age-reversal genius, Professor Ellen Langer. So I feel very confident that the tests are useful. The beauty of them is that you're likely to have everything you need at home already, and, if not, it is all easy to source. I've even made videos of them for you, which you can find on my website (JayneyGoddard.org), so that you can go there for a visual aid to support the text explanations if you find this helpful.

Repeating Every Month to Track Your Progress

Bear in mind that your test results may vary if they are repeated over too short a time frame. This is because we naturally fluctuate for all sorts of reasons: fatigue, stress, hunger and so on. I therefore recommend that you leave a month between tests – and try to ensure that the conditions for each test are the same each time.

It's important to note as many relevant factors as possible, such as time of day, whether you've eaten, if you're very tired and so on, so that you can measure yourself with some degree of accuracy. What we are looking for is an overall trend toward improvement – and when you see this happening, you can be assured that you are rewinding your body clock successfully.

To help you monitor your results, either jot them down in a notebook or, if, like me, you prefer to map your progress more visually with graphs and charts, you can input your data securely and anonymously into the system I have created for you on my website: JayneyGoddard.org. I find it much more motivating when I can see a visual representation of how I'm doing, rather than just looking at lists.

Skin Pinch Test

One of the easiest things you can do to measure your biological age is this Skin Pinch Test, which shows you how elastic your skin is. You will need to have a watch or other timing device at hand.

1. Use the thumb and forefinger of one hand to pinch the skin on the back of your other hand for 5 seconds, then release.
2. Time how long it takes for the skin to settle back into its original form.
3. The longer it takes to go back to normal, the higher your biological age – see the chart below.
4. Repeat this test approximately every month.

The time/age correlation in the Skin Pinch Test is, of course, not definitively accurate, as many factors can affect skin elasticity even temporarily – such as hydration, medications, and even whether you used a hand cream before doing the test – but here is the table that tends to be used to assess results:

Time (seconds)	Biological age (years)
1–2	under 30
3–4	30–44
5–9	45–50
10–15	60
35–55	70
56+	over 70

Do the test three times in a row, calculate the average and make a note of the results in your dedicated place, whether on paper or online, along with a list of specific conditions, such as how hydrated you were and so on.

Balance Test

Balance is another useful indicator of biological age, as well as a good predictor of whether you are prone to having falls. The better your balance, the lower your biological age. So, below is a balance test that was incorporated into the UK's Medical Research Council's paper, "Lifelong Health and Wellbeing: Guidelines for Biomarkers of Healthy Ageing". This closed-eye test can be quite tricky, so it is ideal to have a friend nearby in case you begin to topple. Your friend will also need to time you.

1. Begin by standing barefoot on a stable surface – a hard floor is ideal.
2. Shut your eyes.
3. Bend one knee and lift the foot several centimetres off the ground – there's no need to lift it higher than this.
4. Get your friend to begin to time you.
5. See how long you can hold the position without needing to open your eyes or wobbling.
6. Repeat this three times in total on this leg and then calculate the average time.
7. Now do the same for the left leg.
8. Once you have your averages, check them against the table below.
9. Repeat this test approximately every month.

Balance time (seconds)	*Approximate biological age (years)
4	70
5	65
7	60
8	55
9	50
12	45
16	40
22	30–35
28	25–30

* The age correlation is only approximate, as nothing in ageing is definitive. However, this table will allow you to track your progress.

Vision Test

As we age, we tend to become more long-sighted (presbyopic), which means that we can't see close-up things as well as we used to. This happens because, as we age, our cornea stiffens and is less able to accommodate, or flex, properly in order for us to be able to focus on near objects. Substances called AGEs, which I'll explain in more depth in Chapter 2 (see page 42), are largely responsible for this phenomenon, as they cause the proteins in the cornea to become more rigid. It used to be thought that the progression of presbyopia was unavoidable, but I can attest that although I had started to develop it, it has now reversed, and my near vision is just fine. It goes to show that the damage done by AGEs can be undone! This was an unexpected benefit of implementing and sticking to all the age-reversal approaches I follow personally – and that I share with you in this book.

To do this test, you'll need a ruler and a business card, or another such item with writing on it.

1. Hold the ruler on your cheekbone, sticking out in front of you, horizontal to the floor, and hold the business card at the end of it.
2. Now try to read some of the words on the card at this point. If you can't, find something with slightly larger print and use that.
3. Next, slowly slide the card toward you and make a note of the measurement at which the words on the card start to become blurry.
4. Whether you use a business card or something with larger print, make a note of what you have used, as you'll need it for retesting in approximately a month.

The closer you can get the card to your face and still be able to read it, the better your eyesight and the lower your biological age in this area. See below for a very rough guide to this based on samples of people living in industrialized countries, where it is more likely that they are eating a pro-inflammatory diet loaded with AGE-forming sugars and fats.

Distance between you & ruler (in cm & in)	Approximate age equivalence
Up to 5cm (2in)	Up to 5 years old
Up to 10cm (4in)	Childhood, up to 20 years old
Up to 20cm (8in)	Between early 20s up to circa 42 years old
Up to 40cm (16in)	Early 40s to early/mid-50s
Over 40cm	Mid-50s+

Ruler Drop Reaction Time Test

This is an example of a fitness reaction time test. You'll need a ruler and a partner to assist you. Don't forget that there are videos of all these tests on my website (JayneyGoddard.org) if you would find it helpful to have a more direct visual aid.

1. Sit next to a table so that you can rest the forearm of your dominant side on it; this will stop your arm from moving much during the test.
2. Adjust yourself so that your hand is just overhanging the edge, in a position to hold something, vertically, between thumb and forefinger.
3. Ask your partner to stand in front of you and suspend the ruler vertically between your thumb and index finger so that the zero marking on the ruler is level with them.
4. Without warning, your partner then needs to drop the ruler between your thumb and forefinger, and you need to catch it as fast as you can without moving your forearm from the table.
5. Once you feel comfortable with this practice run, do the same thing 10 times for the real test, making a note of the measurement on the ruler at which you catch it each time. Calculate the average reaction time and make a note of this.
6. Repeat this test approximately every month.

Remember, in order for the test to provide you with genuinely meaningful results, you need to make sure that every time you repeat it, all the conditions are the same. So, for example, the table and chair you sit on must be the same for your arm to be in the same position, and so on.

The actual formula to work out reaction speed equivalents is quite complex and involves calculating the speed of gravitational acceleration and more – so let's not do that! Instead, it's simply best to record your results each time and see how much you can speed up your reaction time over a number of months – with the knowledge that reaction speed is faster in younger people, so it is fair to say that if you are getting faster at the test, there is a good chance that your biological age is reducing.

Flexibility Test

The wider a range of motion you have in your joints, the younger your biological age is in this area. This test, recommended by the Mayo Clinic, a respected non-profit academic medical centre in Minnesota, USA, is a measurement of your flexibility. It is therefore important to do a warm-up prior to attempting it, such as some brisk walking or static stretching.

1. Put a tape measure on the floor, put a mark at the 38cm (15in) point and sit down with your legs outstretched so that your heels align with this 38cm (15in) mark.
2. Reach your arms forward, along the measure, until you can't go any further, and make a note of the measurement at which your hands land.
3. Repeat this stretch two more times and work out your average reach.
4. Repeat this exercise approximately every month.

As we get older, our reach is likely to decrease. According to the Mayo Clinic, a good level of flexibility would be if…

- Men aged up to/around 25 could reach 50cm (19.5in) and women 55cm (21.5in)
- Men aged up to/around 35 could reach 47cm (18.5in) and women 52cm (20.5in)
- Men aged up to/around 45 could reach 44.5cm (17.5in) and women 51cm (20in)

An average reading of greater than 50cm (19.5in) for men and 63cm (25in) for women would be considered excellent.

However, what we are looking for here is simply progression from your own starting point. When you see a progressively longer reach, even if only marginal, you will know that you are starting to successfully rewind your body clock in terms of leg and lower-back flexibility.

Wall Sit Test

You may well "feel the burn" in your thighs when you do this test, as it's a good general strength-building exercise as well as a great way of measuring your biological age regression – particularly in your quadriceps. Don't worry, though, if you're unable to do the exercise for any reason; the other tests will give you a good enough marker of your overall biological age without it.

1. Start by standing against a smooth wall. I like to do this exercise barefoot to minimize any chances of slipping, and on a wall close to a doorframe so that I have something nearby to hold onto and help myself up with should the exercise get too intense.
2. Pressing your back against the wall, slowly slide down it, keeping your feet flat and your shins perpendicular to the floor, and bending your knees until your thighs are at 90 degrees to your shins. Make sure that your knees do not come further forward than your toes.

3. Now time how long you can hold this position before you really feel you have to stop. There's no need to repeat this test several times for an average result like the others. Just repeat it approximately every month.

A round-up of the published results of this test shows that men who can hold this position for more than 102 seconds are considered "excellent". Women receive the same accolade if they can hold for 60 seconds. But, as ever, even if you're nowhere near these times, what you're looking for is an improvement, no matter how small, over time, presuming that you are starting to action a lot of the other recommendations in the book.

Waist Measurements

It's important to note that looking for a reduction in your waist circumference as a biological age marker is only relevant if you are carrying a little extra girth. If you're underweight, then you might expect to see an increase in circumference as you become healthier. So, I'll leave you to be honest with yourself on this one in terms of working out whether you are looking for an increase or decrease. As ever, make sure that you only do the measurement approximately every month, and try to ensure that all the test parameters are the same. As with all the tests, what you are looking for is progress, not perfection. So, even if your initial results are not particularly impressive, it's fine; be gentle with yourself. The whole idea is to see how you improve over time.

Height Measurement

Height may initially seem like an odd thing to measure as a marker of biological age. However, it has been found that people on an age-rewind protocol do tend to get taller if they have previously lost height due to ageing. As we know, people can get shorter as they age, and this is often dismissed as an inevitable part of ageing or as being connected with osteoporosis, which can cause our spinal bones to become more fragile and compact. However, there is more to it than this.

It has been shown that people who believe themselves to be older tend to not walk, stand or sit as upright as they did in their youth. And it follows from this that many people have been found to actually get taller when they feel and believe themselves to be stronger, younger and more independent. The shortening, therefore, hasn't necessarily been a biological problem, but a mindset one. So, as with all the other tests, measure your height every month and see if you notice any difference at all.

Bringing the Results All Together

Once you have done as many of the tests as you can, take a look at all the biological ages that have emerged from the ones that age correlations have been given for. As well as using each age as an indicator of how much you need to focus on that particular area, whether strength, flexibility or whatever else, you might also want to add all the ages together and divide them by the number of different tests you have done, in order to find out your average biological age *overall*.

For example, if you're adding together six ages then divide the total by that number and see how you fare. Again, please don't worry if the result doesn't seem good (as was the case for me when I first did the tests) – simply use this as all the more motivation to get going with the ideas and techniques in this book. If, on the other hand, the result is positive, please don't think that you won't find anything of value for *you* in the book. My hope is that you will still find all kinds of new tidbits of helpful information that you can put into practice in order to maintain, and maybe even further enhance, your current level of vibrancy and youthfulness.

PART I

YOUR REWIND MINDSET

*Understanding Ageing and
Reframing How You View It*

"Ageing is not for sissies."
Bette Davis

We really do have so much more control over how well we age than we realize. And a lot of the science about this is so new that few people are actually aware of it. I have therefore distilled the key research for you in this section – in the hope that you emerge with an increased understanding of the ageing process and a stronger sense of empowerment about just how worthwhile it really is to start following the steps in this book to rewind your body clock naturally. As part of this we will look at:

- The importance of viewing ourselves as holistic beings – with an all-important body–mind connection – in order to get the best results on the Rewind Journey ahead.
- The science behind the ways in which we age, including how developments in the field of epigenetics have now proven how much power we have to alter the course of our own health outcomes.
- The destructive power of inflammation and how, if we can get this under control, we can slow down the biological ageing process.
- The amazing plasticity and adaptability of our brain, including the power of practising both gratitude and compassion to reset our base levels of happiness.
- The incredible power of our mind to affect our body, particularly when it comes to how we deal with stress in our lives and how this affects our capacity to age well.

CHAPTER 1

AGEING: A HOLISTIC PHENOMENON?

The fact that humans are complex individuals means that there are many pieces of the puzzle in understanding how we biologically age. As we have already seen, it is entirely possible for one part of our body, or one aspect of our physiology, to be biologically older than other parts.

A good example of this would be a top-level athlete who is biologically young by all physical fitness measures aside from, for example, her knee joints, which have suffered enormous wear and tear and show signs of inflammation akin to a much older person as her body struggles to repair repeated damage. Similarly, following my life-threatening rheumatoid arthritis flare-up, my bones became fragile and I developed severe osteoporosis. So although, once I was on the road to recovery, things like my body-fat levels were the equivalent of a much younger woman, my bones were biologically ancient.

When we try to understand ageing and the challenges it presents, we therefore need to look at the big picture and view ourselves as "complete biological systems", so that we can get a holistic understanding of exactly how healthy we are overall, and how well we are ageing.

New Paradigms of Health

One of the reasons we need to look to new paradigms to understand ageing is that the existing conventional medical model divides people up into discrete parts. So, if you are suffering concurrently with eczema, type 2 diabetes and arthritis, the conventional model sees these as separate issues, and your GP will refer you to three different specialists: a dermatologist, an endocrinologist and a rheumatologist. This method has

REWIND YOUR BODY CLOCK

much to offer, but it doesn't provide any chance of a permanent solution or cure to chronic health problems, and it definitely doesn't address the premature ageing that chronic diseases cause. While conventional medicine is outstanding at providing life-saving solutions in emergency situations, we also have to acknowledge that looking to the current medical system for solutions to unhealthy ageing probably isn't the wisest move, as the medical model doesn't yet fully embrace the immense impact that every aspect of lifestyle has upon our health and wellbeing.

Embracing a Lifestyle Approach

Happily, there is some light on the horizon, in that increasing numbers of doctors and health practitioners are starting to embrace what is called a "Lifestyle Medicine" approach. This is the long-overdue acknowledgement from both scientists and the medical profession that a holistic approach, integrating a wide range of therapies, is necessary if we are to become healthier overall, and live longer, with enhanced health-spans.

This is the same approach we have been taking in complementary medicine and natural healthcare for aeons, but even afficionados at Harvard Medical School are now stating that the most important lifestyle change to avoid and combat dementia (including Alzheimer's and Parkinson's diseases) is to adopt a plant-based, wholefood diet – one of the core tenets of this book.

The Royal Society of Medicine – who tend to be even more conservative than Harvard Medical School – only recently had a symposium on plant-based nutrition to combat chronic disease, and they also ran another symposium on gut health and the microbiome (read more about this in Chapter 7) as they relate to our mental health. This is unprecedented in medicine and it's great to see an admission, at last, that we human beings are holistic entities, that everything is connected, and that it is no longer viable for medicine to think of us in terms of disparate parts.

A Wellbeing Revolution

A good example of science being able to distil things down to just its most effective part, or parts, can be found in the work of Dr Herbert Benson, who runs the Benson-Henry Institute at Harvard Medical School and is considered to be the "father" of what is called Mind/Body Medicine – another new model of medicine that helps us to understand how we function as whole human beings.

Rewind Insight: You might well be wondering at this stage what the difference is between Lifestyle Medicine, Mind/Body Medicine and complementary medicine, so here is a quick overview for you:

- Lifestyle Medicine is an approach that believes that we humans benefit from a holistic approach – so that what we eat, think, how we exercise, our social relationships, our spirituality and our connection to the world at large are all deemed to be important to our wellbeing.
- Mind/Body Medicine can be viewed as an important part of Lifestyle Medicine as it is the study and practice of the way that our mind and body relate to each other, how one influences the other and vice versa.
- And complementary medicine comprises all of the healthcare disciplines that are not a part of conventional medicine, such as nutrition, massage, acupuncture, hypnosis, homeopathy, herbal medicine and many more. The commonality is that these disciplines all aim to take the *whole* patient into consideration – mentally, emotionally, physically and spiritually.

Dr Benson made enormous breakthroughs in wellbeing science, including an observation that there were huge health benefits for people who meditated regularly. Until that point in the 1960s, the meditators who had been studied the most were practising Transcendental Meditation (TM). In terms of science, the benefits of this type of meditation were proving to be undeniable. However, because TM is just one aspect of a whole, wider approach to life, it was difficult to ascertain exactly why TM worked so well.

Was it the act of simply sitting still for 20 minutes, twice a day, that resulted in the health-giving effects? Was it the repetition of a unique personal mantra bestowed by a teacher? Or was it something altogether different? There were so many variables, or "confounding matters" to use the scientific term, which could have been the reason. However, Dr Benson and his colleagues worked to tease out answers and went on to formulate a secular approach to meditation which works just as well, but which has no allegiance to a particular spiritual or religious organization. Dr Benson essentially demystified the process of meditation for health benefits, simplifying it right down to the most effective part, which turned out to be what he called the "Relaxation Response" – a method of calming the breath and mind, building resilience to stressors and creating profound positive changes to health in all respects (see page 62 for more on this).

I strongly believe that future generations will look back on breakthroughs like this, and on this period of enhanced scientific curiosity about holistic health, as the seat of a wellbeing revolution. And by buying books like this and following the guidance in them, you are part of this revolution.

So, in the spirit of this, let's move on now to a chapter in which you have the chance to learn a little about the science behind the process of ageing. This chapter might can get a little in-depth – and maybe even geeky at times – but if you can bear with me, you will benefit, as it will give you more insight into just why the recommendations in this book will support you greatly in attaining your health, healing and happiness goals. As a result, you'll feel much more empowered in your Rewind Journey, and making the best choices for your health will become second nature, as you'll know exactly what works and why.

CHAPTER 2

THE SCIENCE OF AGEING

The information in this chapter will help you understand what is actually happening in our bodies as we age, and how much power we really have over this process. It is so much easier to make ongoing, sustainable change toward rewinding your body clock if you really understand the reasons that these changes are recommended – and the science behind them.

The science here heralds from some of the finest scientific brains around and is the basis and springboard for many of the theories and practices that I share with you throughout the book, so I do hope you find it both interesting and enlightening.

Key Theories of Ageing

There are a lot of theories about ageing (literally hundreds!), but for the purposes of this book I have chosen the following four, given that they are used so widely across anti-ageing and gerontology research and therefore feel most relevant to this book:

- Oxidization
- Glycation and AGEs
- Telomere Shortening
- The Hayflick Theory

Oxidization

The oxidization theory was developed by Denham Harman, MD, at the University of Nebraska in 1956. It is based on the idea that damage occurs when healthy tissue is attacked by unstable molecules called free radicals. It is known that diet, lifestyle, radiation and drugs, including tobacco and alcohol, are accelerators of free-radical production within the body.

Thankfully, free radicals can be transformed by free-radical scavengers known as antioxidants. Substances such as beta carotene, vitamins C and E, olive leaf extract, açaï, grape seed extract and all fruits and vegetables contain powerful antioxidants, so can help in the quest for more positive ageing.

Glycation

The Glycation Theory of Ageing, also known as the Cross-Linking Theory of Ageing, suggests that the excessive binding of glucose to protein in the presence of oxygen causes various problems. This cross-linking is also known as Advanced Glycation End-Products, or AGEs.

Why, you might ask, should we care about the cross-linking of proteins? First, let's look at proteins, what they are and where they are found. Proteins are made up of amino acids and these are essential for life because they serve two vital roles:

1. Structure: Collagen makes up approximately one third of your body's total protein. Collagen is found in organs, muscles, skin and vascular structures including veins, arteries and capillaries, and it provides all of these with the ability to be elastic and responsive.
2. Enzyme activity: Proteins support enzyme activity that enables all life-sustaining biochemical reactions to happen in your body.

Sugar provides energy for your cells, and when this process is working well, proteins and sugars work together without inflicting damage. However, once sugars bind to proteins (the process of glycation), the protein becomes compromised, can't work as efficiently and becomes stiff. This can lead to all sorts of problems, including hardening of the arteries, senile cataracts, kidney disease and the appearance of tough, leathery, wrinkled and yellow skin. AGEs may also be responsible for cardiac enlargement, which can lead to an increased likelihood of heart disease. In fact, the latest research shows that glycation may be more sinister than originally believed; it is thought that sugars binding to our DNA can potentially cause damage that could lead to malfunctioning cells and cancer.

Type 2 diabetes is often viewed as a form of accelerated ageing, with the imbalance of insulin and glucose intolerance leading to serious health problems that have been dubbed "Syndrome X". Type 1 diabetes is an altogether different health issue, predominantly caused by an autoimmune problem, which results in the destruction of the insulin-producing beta cells in the pancreas. Despite the differences in the causes of both, the end results are similar in that they manifest as a body unable to process glucose properly. In fact, because of chronically elevated blood sugars, diabetics of both types have two to three times more cross-linked proteins than healthy people, and this causes them to age faster.

The very latest research is starting to suggest that Alzheimer's disease could feasibly be called type 3 diabetes, as it could be caused by the detrimental effect of sugars cross-linking with proteins in the brain, which results in a variety of serious neurological problems.

Telomere Shortening

Telomeres are the end sections of our chromosomes and can be likened to the plastic ends of shoelaces, called aglets. Discovered by the Nobel Prize-winning scientist Elizabeth Blackburn, telomeres are, in fact, sequences of nucleic acids that extend from the ends of chromosomes, and they shorten every time a cell divides. This shortening is believed to lead to cellular damage, as each time a cell divides, it duplicates itself a little worse than the time before – a bit like taking a photocopy of a photocopy and so on – eventually leading to cellular dysfunction, ageing and, ultimately, cell death.

One of the key elements in rebuilding shrinking telomeres is the enzyme telomerase, also discovered by Professor Blackburn. Although so far only found in "germ" cells (ovary and sperm) and cancer cells, telomerase appears to repair and replace telomeres, helping to re-regulate the clock that controls the lifespan of dividing cells, known as the Hayflick Limit, which we'll come to a bit later in this chapter (see page 44).

As touched on earlier in this book, it's actually possible these days to have your telomeres measured, but it's an expensive procedure, and it would be wise to approach the accuracy of results with caution. Even the few specialists offering telomere age testing are cautious about how accurate the tests are if looked at in isolation. Current research on different parts of our bodies ageing at different rates means that telomere length in different areas is likely to vary, rendering any specific telomere testing redundant if people are trying to ascertain their *overall* biological age. However, measuring telomeres can still be useful in more experimental settings, as similar samples can be taken from groups of people over time, which can provide data, such as the average speed at which telomeres shorten. Faster shortening means that a person is ageing more rapidly within the specific parameters of that particular test.

There are no conventional medical interventions that can preserve the length of telomeres, and only one supplement derived from a plant is beginning to show promise, but it is too early to tell just how effective this will be in the absence of making any lifestyle changes. Scientists also question whether adding telomerase from external sources could provoke the development of cancer – which is why it is best to improve the production of your own, endogenous, telomerase. However, there is one proven way of stopping the shortening of telomeres and re-growing them, and that is lifestyle modification, including everything from eating youth-promoting foods and doing regular moderate exercise to meditation and developing greater resilience toward stress. In fact, everything that we will cover in this book!

The Hayflick Theory

In 1961, Dr Leonard Hayflick theorized that human cells' ability to divide is limited to approximately 50 times, after which they simply stop dividing and subsequently die. Dr Hayflick showed that nutrition has an important effect on cells, with overfed cells dividing and eventually dying off much faster than underfed cells.

From research started in the 1930s, we know that calorie restriction in animals significantly increases their lifespan. So might this be due to reduced free-radical activity and therefore less cellular damage? Or could it be that insulin and glucose damage is not as prevalent compared to that in overfed animals? Is there an alteration in their genetic expression that prevents the development of the diseases of ageing? Maybe the answer lies in a combination of all these factors as well as others.

Whatever the answer, a theory known as the Hayflick Limit indicates the need to slow the rate of cell division if we want to live long, healthy lives. And the way to do this, according to current scientific consensus, is by adhering to a calorie-poor but nutrient-rich diet. This way of eating, as we shall see in Chapter 6, also helps to preserve our telomere length, enabling us to lengthen our health-span as well as our lifespan.

Epigenetics

Another important component to consider when thinking about anti-ageing is the relatively new field of epigenetics – the study of how our genes express themselves, and how internal and external influences can switch on or off certain genes.

Many people believe that they are completely defined, limited, even imprisoned, by the deck of genetic cards they were dealt at birth. You often hear people exclaim that because their parents or grandparents had diabetes, heart disease or some form of cancer, they too are likely to develop the same problems. This fear is magnified when people discover that they have some genetic predisposition, like the BRCA gene in women that may cause them to develop breast cancer or ovarian cancer. These women can feel as if they have no choice but to opt for medical intervention that might, at best, compromise their health and, at worst, coerce them into surrendering vital body parts to surgical mutilation for fear of what may happen in the future.

Recent discoveries in epigenetics clearly demonstrate that we are most definitely *not* completely at the mercy of our genetic inheritance! Indeed, we can take simple and sustainable steps to protect our own health.

Your genetic blueprint can, of course, predispose you to any number of positive and negative conditions and cellular changes, but the key word here is "predispose". Your individual genetic blueprint is malleable, so what you choose to do, and the healthy or unhealthy choices you make on a daily basis in your life, will go a long way to determining how your genetic predisposition expresses itself.

In 2007, Dr Dean Ornish and his team conducted a study on men with slow-growing prostate cancer who had decided not to have conventional treatment but had opted instead for monitoring of the condition to see if changes occurred. They were put on a plant-based, vegan, wholefood, low-fat diet, asked to exercise, and taught meditation and mindfulness techniques. As with previous studies where lifestyle interventions had been introduced, the men experienced significant improvements in weight, reduced abdominal obesity, improved blood pressure and blood lipid profile. However, what was really exciting was that when Dr Ornish and his colleagues analysed the men's gene expression (in this case expression means how the genes actually function), it was discovered that 48 genes were up-regulated (more active), while 453 were down-regulated (less active) by the end of the experiment. The analysis of the particular genetic expressions that changed during the experiment showed that the biological processes that were the most important in suppressing the development of tumours were the most active. Ornish and his colleagues concluded from this that "Intensive nutrition and lifestyle changes may modulate gene expression in the prostate."

We therefore really do have more power than we often think when it comes to our own health and ageing process if we can only get ourselves to commit to making strong holistic health decisions in life and consistently following through on them.

CHAPTER 3

UNDERSTANDING INFLAMMATION

Inflammation has been proven to underlie every condition that we associate with ageing right across the board, from wrinkles to lifestyle-related cancers, right through to Alzheimer's disease. In fact, many of the leading health experts now use the term "inflammaging" to describe the undeniable link between ageing and inflammation. Understanding inflammation as part of ageing is therefore incredibly important – and getting to grips with just how much control you have over it is vital.

The damage that inflammation can cause is devastating – but I want you to know that you are most definitely not at the mercy of this problem, as chronic inflammation can be halted quickly using the lifestyle approaches in this book. Once you make these changes, you'll start feeling measurably younger, happier and fitter in both body and mind.

So What Exactly Is Inflammation?

Inflammation is an immune response that your body mounts in order to deal with anything that your body perceives as an "attack" that could result in harm. Usually this rapid, short-term or "acute" response is appropriate and protects us. For example, if you sprain your ankle, your body will produce a range of symptoms including pain, heat and swelling. This is appropriate as it is, after all, imperative that you don't walk on the ankle and damage it further. Similarly, if you get a cold or flu, your immune system will respond by producing a variety of chemical messengers (cytokines) that fight pathogens (or "invaders") in various ways, including helping to raise your temperature to kill viruses etc. through heat – making you feel ill and forcing you to rest to get better.

Chronic inflammation, however, is a completely different ball game. It has dire health consequences. An immune response that lasts for a long time, it is linked to obesity, fat around the middle, depression, cancers, heart disease, asthma, the complications of diabetes (types 1 and 2), neurological diseases including Alzheimer's and Parkinson's, arthritis of all forms, and it also increases our sensitivity to pain, accelerates free-radical damage and suppresses healthy immune function, rendering us more susceptible to both acute and chronic diseases.

Many people think of inflammation as purely a physical problem. But, in reality, it is so connected to our psyche (it has now been proven to be a cause of depression, for example), that I feel it is crucial to include it upfront here in order to add it to your growing knowledge of the jigsaw puzzle that is the ageing process, in order to help enhance your overall Rewind mindset.

Treating Inflammation

As I described in the Introduction, I know from my own experience just how devastating runaway chronic inflammation is and how costly it can be from an ageing perspective, as I aged dramatically when I went through my health meltdown (which I now know was caused by totally out-of-control inflammation, related to a huge rheumatoid arthritis flare-up).

You see, all the diseases we associate with ageing, and even biological ageing itself, are dramatically accelerated when our bodies are producing a chronic inflammatory response.

However, unfortunately, there is nothing that conventional medicine has to offer to deal with chronic inflammation from a "curative" standpoint. All that anti-inflammatories, from basic aspirin and ibuprofen right up to intensive courses of steroids, do is aim to simply relieve symptoms in order to make life temporarily more bearable for the patient: a Band-Aid approach. And over-the-counter Non-Steroidal Anti-Inflammatory Drugs (NSAIDs) can cause a range of serious health problems, as well as dramatically increasing our risk of developing cardiovascular issues. Severe side effects from these drugs are, in fact, one of the main reasons for non-traumatic hospital admissions. To illustrate just how dangerous such over-the-counter anti-inflammatories can be, an article in the *British Journal of General Practice* explained that NSAIDs are responsible for more deaths in the UK than road traffic accidents, and twice as many deaths as from asthma or cervical cancer, per annum.

Living an Anti-Inflammatory Lifestyle

Everybody living in industrialized, "Westernized" nations – with no exceptions – would therefore benefit tremendously from cultivating an anti-inflammatory lifestyle in the first place. This would support us in being healthy and balanced in both body and mind, regardless of the stresses and strains of modern living. And the encouraging news is that chronic inflammation has been proven to respond both positively and rapidly to positive lifestyle measures, including following a plant-based, wholefood, anti-inflammatory diet (see Chapter 6 for more on this), although diet is, of course, just part of the equation. Other measures include everything from appropriate exercise and building strong personal relationships, to spending time in nature and getting good sleep, all of which are covered in this book.

Monitoring Inflammation

In order to begin to deal with any *chronic* inflammation in your system, it's important to recognize and address any longstanding illnesses or signs of premature ageing that you have. So, if you have a particular health issue that hasn't resolved itself naturally, the first step is to get it checked out by your doctor in order to rule out anything that can be successfully treated using conventional medical approaches. However, given that *all* chronic diseases and their symptoms, as well as a lot of signs of premature ageing, have uncontrolled inflammation as a main component, the only way to *fully* deal with these conditions and return to a state of good health is by harnessing lifestyle approaches like the Rewind ones in this book, too. Remember, you have so much more control over how you age than you probably realize – all the choices you make today will predict your health tomorrow.

If you want to get a measure of how much your body is currently affected by inflammation, you could ask your doctor for a blood test to ascertain your C Reactive Protein (CRP) levels, as this is one of the most important markers used to detect inflammation. To get the most accurate test, request a High-Sensitivity CRP (hs-CRP) test. CRP can change very rapidly, though, so it is good to get tested every month to six weeks initially, as you are looking for overall trends.

Monitoring and eradicating chronic, out-of-control inflammation really is one of the keys to feeling and looking better, healthier, happier and younger; as we mentioned earlier, there's a proven connection between chronic inflammation and depression, for example.

The Benefits of Reducing Inflammation

With inflammation under control, you'll soon find yourself sleeping better, having more energy, feeling more motivated as well as enjoying stronger brain power, an improved libido and better body composition. You're particularly likely to benefit from more muscle and less fat – especially reduced fat around the middle and less toxic "visceral fat" around the organs, which could otherwise drive inflammation, thus potentially keeping you in a vicious circle.

CHAPTER 4

THE NEUROBIOLOGY OF HAPPINESS

In this chapter, I'm going to share with you information and techniques on the power of training yourself to develop a more positive outlook on life in order to stay in optimal mental and emotional shape. As well as making you feel generally better on a day-to-day basis, this has now been proven to reduce your risks of developing many of the chronic diseases we associate with ageing.

Brain Flux

Neurobiology is the study of the biology, structure and function of the brain. Until recently, scientists believed that the brain was a fairly fixed entity and that the only change it underwent was a mass die-off of cells after the age of 40. Happily, however, the relatively new understanding of the concept of neuroplasticity – one of the great buzzwords of the moment – has led us to understand that when we have new thoughts and feelings, our brain actually adapts as a result of them.

Our brain is, in fact, therefore in a constant state of flux, ever adapting, growing new connections and evolving in order to facilitate function. It can even physically change shape as well as the way that it functions. And if someone is unlucky enough to suffer damage to a particular part of the brain, and a specific physical, emotional or cognitive function is compromised, there is a strong possibility that other parts of the brain not normally associated with that function will take over and adapt to enable them to regain the lost function. Hence you may have heard stories of what seem like miraculous recoveries from severe injuries, strokes and the like. This is neuroplasticity at work in all its brilliance.

Another important brain-science phenomenon that's particularly relevant in the context of this book is the notion that "synapses that fire together wire together". What on earth am I talking about, you might well be asking? There is a gap or cleft between neurons (nerve cells) called a "synaptic cleft", and each time we have a thought or feeling, a chemical is diffused across this gap, building a bridge and thus passing along the relevant information that you are experiencing – so that the neurons can be said to "fire together".

Now, here's the incredible thing. Every time this chemical is diffused across the synaptic cleft, your neural pathways can be said to bond more strongly or "wire together". And this means, in essence, that your brain is adapting so that the same thought or feeling can be more readily experienced the next time.

The Importance of Positive Thoughts

Given that your brain is constantly reshaping itself with every thought, it's crucial to realize that any recurring thoughts we have will cause certain sets of synapses to bond or "wire" together significantly more strongly. And the strongest bonds (that is to say the ones we can access more readily given we have primed our brains to react that way) become our default personality. Essentially, the subjects we think about most frequently and the emotions we feel most frequently become our hardwired set point.

This means that if we often do things we enjoy, spend time with people who lift our spirits and generally think happy thoughts, the bridges between the neurons that enable the happy thoughts will grow stronger and we will tend toward feeling more positive and vibrant as a result. If, on the other hand, we focus on the negative in our lives, associate a lot with people who bring us down and think unhappy thoughts, the bridges between *those* neurons will get stronger, allowing negative, unhealthy patterns to thrive and become our "norm", which will lead to a less positive ageing experience. Looking at things from this perspective, it's certainly easy to see why it makes sense to choose our thoughts wisely, as recurring negative thought patterns can, rather scarily, genuinely lead to dissatisfaction, depression, premature ageing and feeling unwell.

Given what we know about how the brain shapes itself to assist and facilitate our most frequent thoughts and feelings, it makes perfect sense to create a setpoint within ourselves that is optimally healthy. Especially as we also know from the science of psychoneuroimmunology that ongoing, repeated negative emotions, such as fear, anger, jealousy, guilt, lack of gratitude, and a focus on complaining and negativity, provoke the release of a slew of neurotransmitters or chemical messengers that directly cause chronic inflammation. And, as we explored in Chapter 3 (on inflammation), chronic inflammation is at the root of all the diseases we often mistakenly attribute to ageing and decline.

The Art of Acceptance and Training Our Thoughts

So how on earth can we shift from simply reacting to situations any old way that emerges (whether positive or negative at the time) to actively choosing more regular positive thoughts and responses that produce life-affirming emotions, such as love, happiness, awe, gratitude, compassion and kindness – feelings that will lead to mental, emotional, physical and spiritual wellbeing? After all, life is unpredictable and tends to throw us the occasional curve ball, making it a challenge to keep thinking positively.

One of the most crucial steps we can take on this journey is making an active choice to *accept* and love whatever comes our way with an optimistic outlook – viewing life events, whether seemingly good or bad, as life lessons that we are OK with and will get through. Two actions that will help enormously with this are:

- Cultivating more gratitude for what we have in life (rather than allowing ourselves to focus on what we don't have)
- Cultivating more loving kindness for both ourselves and others (rather than constantly judging and harshly criticizing)

I therefore include information and guidance on two practices in the pages that follow to help you achieve both these things. Please know that I'm not talking about a "Pollyanna" outlook here – I'm by no means suggesting that we deny the existence of the harder things in life or that we just pretend things are all rosy. In fact, the approach I'm advocating fully acknowledges the tougher aspects of life; it simply encourages us to choose and craft our responses to them and is therefore one of the most important things we can do to enhance our wellbeing.

By starting to choose our thoughts and feelings with more awareness, gratitude and compassion, we will create strong, loving synapses that will wire preferentially so that our personality setpoint becomes a more positive, vibrant one than before, with innate mental, emotional and spiritual strength and resilience. We should therefore soon find that our world feels like a happier, healthier, more beautiful place in which to live as a result.

The Power of Gratitude

Dr Robert Emmons, the world's leading gratitude researcher, describes gratitude as the "felt sense of wonder, thankfulness and appreciation for life". It's likely that we all utter fleeting expressions of gratitude in our daily lives, such as thanking someone when they make us a cup of tea or hold a door open for us, and these are nice things. However, an active practice of really connecting to profound gratitude goes much deeper.

One of the most fascinating discoveries to emerge from the field of positive psychology in terms of how human beings flourish is that the regular and deliberate practice of deep gratitude can create significant relief from stress and great improvements in happiness, motivation, optimism, energy levels, quality of sleep and quality of life.

I therefore present opposite a core gratitude practice that you can come back to at any time throughout your Rewind Journey to help ensure a grateful frame of mind. By doing this any time you feel yourself losing focus or positivity, you'll maintain the best possible mindset to recognize the benefits starting to emerge from all the positive steps you are taking as a result of reading this book.

The Power of Loving Kindness

Another highly effective way of rewiring your mind to start living with more positive thoughts is the regular practice of a simple but powerful meditation from the Buddhist tradition called a "Metta Meditation", which centres around the concepts of loving kindness and compassion. This encourages you not only to accept and love yourself and your loved ones, complete with all their flaws, but also to accept everything and everyone beyond this too, even people or circumstances that may cause you angst.

You'll find a step-by-step version of this transformational practice overleaf (on page 56) to use at any time during your Rewind Journey. Among its many benefits, it will help prevent you from being too harsh on yourself as you work toward your goals. You will also find a recording of a variation of this Loving Kindness, or Metta, Meditation at JayneyGoddard.org.

Having qualified as a Zen meditation teacher in 2014, I'm aware that many people are keen to practise meditation but are put off by the amount of time they think is needed for it. However, it was recently reported in the *International Journal of Geriatric Psychiatry* by a team of researchers including both Elizabeth Blackburn and Elissa Epel that dramatic changes to our health and wellbeing can occur with just 12 minutes of meditation per day, which means that it's now easier than ever to reap the benefits.

REWIND ANCHOR PRACTICE
Cultivate Gratitude

When we are in a grateful frame of mind, things seem both more possible and more positive. It is therefore immensely useful when aiming to rewind your body clock to make a concerted effort to develop an "attitude of gratitude" in your day-to-day life. Below are some simple ways to do this:

- Take a moment now and again throughout each day to recognize the good things and count your blessings.
- Keep a journal in which you write down three things at the end of each day for which you are grateful.
- Take time out now and again to write a letter of gratitude to someone important to you; this can be particularly useful if you're feeling low.

In case you find it difficult at times to identify everyday things that you feel grateful for, here follows a list of questions for you to ask yourself in order to help you find more focus. Feel free to either answer each one in your head or jot down the answers on a piece of paper or in your journal.

- What basic necessities in life are you grateful for?
- Do you have any favourite childhood memories?
- What are your best memories about an old friend, or a pet?
- What is beautiful about your immediate environment?
- What do you feel happy about having accomplished in your life?
- What makes your life easier?
- What is the best thing that happened this week, this month or this year?
- Can you recall a happy memory from five years ago?
- What is the most beautiful sound you can hear right now?
- What is your most cherished dream for the future?

The key with all these practices is to really try to *feel* into the gratitude. After a week or so, you might want to continue doing the exercise daily, or you might prefer to reduce it to something like a couple of times a week. It's important to stop it from becoming boring, because if you start resenting the process, it will be counterproductive. So choose what is best for you. It can be very uplifting to look back over a gratitude journal and feel inspired as you see all the lovely things you have written about.

REWIND ANCHOR PRACTICE
Loving Kindness Meditation

Many studies have proven that regular practice of a loving kindness meditation technique such as the one below is linked to greater, more consistent feelings of happiness, which will help you no end on your Rewind Journey.

1. Sit comfortably, somewhere quiet, with your eyes closed, and say silently to yourself something along the lines of "May I be healthy. May I be happy. May I be safe from harm." Spend at least 3 minutes (or more if you have it) directing these kind thoughts toward yourself.

2. Next, choose someone you feel close to and thankful for – someone who has been good to you – and direct the same kind words, and therefore thoughts, toward them for the same amount of time: "May X be healthy. May X be happy. May X be safe from harm."

3. The next step is to bring to mind a neutral person – somebody you neither like nor dislike – and direct the same thoughts toward them for the same amount of time again. This can feel quite difficult at first, as we often very quickly formulate subconscious opinions about others, but it could be someone you see as you go about your daily business, whether a shop worker, a co-commuter or a passerby: "May Y be healthy. May Y be happy. May Y be safe from harm."

4. Next, bring to mind a person you're having a difficult time with or who you don't like, and direct the same words and thoughts toward them for the same amount of time again: "May Z be healthy. May Z be happy. May Z be safe from harm."

5. Lastly, take a little time to send the same loving thoughts out universally by saying: "May all beings everywhere be healthy. May all beings everywhere be happy. May all beings everywhere be safe from harm."

6. Once you have finished, sit quietly for a minute or two, basking in the feelings of love that you have just generated, before opening your eyes and resuming normal activities.

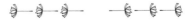

CHAPTER 5

STRESS RESPONSE MANAGEMENT AND THE POWER OF THE MIND

Stress is one of the most aggressively ageing lifestyle factors there is. And while, as we all know, life happens, and stressful events occur whether we want them to or not, happily, we all have a lot more control over how we choose to *respond* to stress than we often realize. As such, we can take steps that will have a hugely positive impact on our mindset and therefore on our health, happiness and the speed at which we biologically age.

You'll notice that I don't talk about "stress reduction" or "stress management" in this chapter, as there's often little we can do about events that unfold. Instead, I prefer the term "stress response management" and the idea of building as much resilience as possible to stress, so that when we are exposed to stressors, the effect they have on us is greatly reduced.

So, let's begin by looking at some of the studies that illustrate just how harmful poor, pessimistic responses to stressful life events can be, and then we'll look at the life-extending and health-supporting effects of optimism and some techniques that we can practise to encourage this.

How Stress Shortens Life

We're starting to understand the relationship between stress, the development of chronic diseases and premature death. Chronic psychological stress is associated with accelerated shortening of telomeres, which causes the chromosomes to "die" faster (see also Chapter 2).

A recent fascinating study compared 39 healthy, premenopausal women who looked after a child who had a severe chronic illness against 19 mothers of a similar age who had healthy children. Both sets of women completed a questionnaire about their stress levels and their telomere length was measured in their blood samples. The mothers who cared for the seriously ill children had much shorter telomeres. In fact, the mothers who had the highest levels of stress had an average of a 550-unit telomere shortening versus the mothers of healthy children. What this means in real terms is that the highly stressed mothers were, biologically speaking, 9–17 years older than the mothers of the healthy children. Similar premature-ageing results have also been seen in carers of people with Alzheimer's. Accelerated ageing is just one of the reasons it is so important for our society to develop more resources to care for carers, with an emphasis on helping them to integrate healthy lifestyle factors into their lives.

Optimism Increases Lifespan

On a happier note, studies have also proven that having a positive attitude improves your responses to daily stress, which can potentially increase both your health-span and lifespan. One of the best ways of creating a more optimistic outlook is by embracing the philosophy of "It's not what happens to me; it's what I make of it."

Researchers in the Netherlands found that older men and women who had optimistic personalities were less likely to die over a nine-year period than those with pessimistic outlooks. An attitude of optimism seems to be particularly important in protecting against heart disease: optimists in the study were 77 per cent less likely to die of a heart attack, stroke or other cardiovascular cause than the most pessimistic group. And this was the case regardless of factors such as age, weight, smoking and whether the participants had cardiovascular or other chronic diseases at the start.

Another study of people aged 50 and over, who were followed for an average of 23 years and who believed that they had a positive attitude toward ageing, lived an average of more than seven years longer than those who had a more negative view of getting older.

It has also been proven as important to keep working as long as possible if you want to live longer and more healthily. A report in the *British Medical Journal* showed that people who retired later tend to live longer. (On a personal note, I'm fascinated by what the mindset factors are that can help us to live a healthy long life, so I have a bit of a habit of cornering healthy-looking elderly people to find out their secrets! I have to say that most people I have talked with have a common mindset: they are either still working into advanced age, or they volunteer. I've also noticed that they make a point of getting up each day and getting neatly, attractively or smartly dressed. These elderly people also seem to be very interested in wellness topics and have conscious healthy-eating strategies. Clearly, these are just my observations, so this is merely anecdotal – but to me, these factors seem like no coincidence.)

My Experience of Positive Visualization

When I got very ill, as explained on page 3, my inflammation was so out of control that I became cachexic – which means my body was actually consuming my tissues for fuel, including muscle tissue. I therefore lost a lot of weight and couldn't move. My muscle wastage was so extreme that my brain had "forgotten" how to move my body and I was locked, immobile, into a foetal position. I had been told by my consultant that I'd never walk, or even stand, again. He actually said to me, "Just face it, you are always going to be chair-shaped" – referring to my wheelchair! The outlook was grim and the only conventional medication offered to me was chemotherapy to kill off my immune system and hopefully give me some relief from this relentless immune attack. So, as you can imagine, this left me feeling pretty down and, in certain moments, deeply pessimistic.

However, ultimately, I wasn't willing to just accept this fate, and I knew enough about my own body to realize that, what with already being so gravely ill and underweight, putting a highly toxic drug into my system was probably not the cleverest idea. I therefore did some soul searching and worked out that I needed to somehow pay more attention to the mind–body connection explained in the Introduction. Given that I had no muscle left to speak of, I realized I had to harness my mind to "communicate" more positively with my body, so that I could perhaps encourage my immune system to calm down and stop attacking me. I therefore decided to play ballet music and simply *imagine* myself dancing, given that I couldn't do it physically. Dancing was something I could relate to on every level, having previously been a professional dancer.

As I started this, I became determined to not just live, but to really get better and thrive. And the key is that I *totally* believed that this would be achievable. Of course, I also made sure that all other aspects of my lifestyle were supporting the positive visualization, from optimal nutrition to adequate levels of gratitude, meditation and stress-response management. And, little by little, I started to get better: firstly the pain and inflammation subsided; then a few muscle fibres started twitching; and, eventually, I managed to regain full use of my body! I share this story with you to show that, even in the worst situations, we can harness the power of our minds to gain strength, heal and potentially get better.

The Proven Power of Visualization

Many scientific studies have also been done that back up my *personal* experience of it being possible to make improvements in strength and fitness without lifting a finger – and instead by exercising just the mind!

One of my favourites is one in which the researchers measured strength improvements in three different groups of people: the first group continued with their normal daily routine as before; the second group did two weeks of highly focused strength training for one specific muscle, three times a week; and the third group listened to recordings that helped them to *imagine* doing the same workout as the exercising group three times a week – but they did no physical exercise. The results were astonishing: predictably, the control group saw no improvement in strength; the exercise group saw a 28 per cent gain in strength; but the group who *visualized* exercising experienced nearly the same gains in strength as the exercise group, at 24 per cent! It's pretty astonishing stuff.

The mind has also been proven to have the power to make you slimmer! In a Harvard study, housekeeping staff in a major hotel were told that the work they did on a daily basis equalled the amount of exercise needed to be fit and healthy. They made no changes in behaviour; they just kept on doing their job with this new belief in place. Four weeks later, the housekeepers had lost weight, lowered their blood pressure, had improved body-fat percentage, developed a healthier waist–hip ratio and a better BMI. A similar group of housekeepers (the control group) who had not been led to believe their job qualified as exercise saw none of these changes.

All in all, then, the power of the mind is really pretty incredible. So much so that many top sports people use visualization techniques to mentally rehearse their events before they compete with great success.

Of course, this doesn't mean for one minute that visualization is *all* you should do. However, it is *particularly* useful to incorporate positive visualization techniques into the recovery programme of anyone who is injured or immobilized. And positive visualization is also extremely helpful at any time for fit and healthy people who simply want a boost on their Rewind Journey, so see the page opposite for some guidance on this.

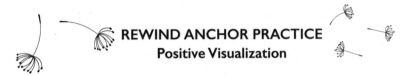

REWIND ANCHOR PRACTICE
Positive Visualization

When I was ill and unable to physically exercise to keep myself strong, I used a ballet dancing visualization to rewind my body clock. However, it's vital that you choose your own image when using positive visualization, depending on what your main aims are, as well as the activities and exercises you have the most positive associations with.

Consider what the most effective visualization for you might be given your current circumstances. What would you most like to achieve from using visualization? For example, more strength? More mobility? More positivity? More energy? Or something other than these? And which activity, or activities, do you feel would give you what you need based on your previous experience? Then set aside some regular time to imagine yourself doing this.

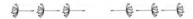

The Power of Relaxation

I learned about the "Relaxation Response" at Harvard Medical School, directly from the man who created it, Dr Herbert Benson. According to Dr Benson, one of the most valuable things we can do in life is learn deep relaxation – making an effort to spend some time every day quietening our minds to help cope with stress and create enhanced wellbeing, which, as we know by now, can dramatically help with how well we age.

There are many methods to bring about variations of the Relaxation Response, including visualization, meditation, progressive muscle relaxation, energy healing and all sorts of holistic practices and treatments from yoga and tai chi to acupuncture and massage. See overleaf for my choice of guidance for you in this book. You will also find an instructional recording on my website (JayneyGoddard.org), as it is often so much easier to listen to someone talking you through an exercise than to read it and try to remember what you're supposed to be doing.

REWIND ANCHOR PRACTICE
The Relaxation Response

This exercise can be done at any time during your Rewind Journey that you feel like stress is taking over and you need some time out to recalibrate in order to get the most from the other techniques in the book.

In an ideal world, however, it would be best to practise it once or twice daily for 10 to 20 minutes at a time. Avoid doing it within two hours after eating, though, as the digestive process intereferes with the Relaxation Response. And it's best not to use a timer, so that you start getting used to instinctively judging your timings.

1. Sit comfortably somewhere quiet and close your eyes.
2. Starting at your feet, allow them to deeply relax as much as possible, letting go of any tension you may find there.
3. Slowly work your way up your entire body – from your shins, knees and thighs, right up to your head and face – checking in with each part and releasing any tension as you go. Take your time to do this so that you really feel each part of your body relaxing deeply.
4. As you focus on releasing tension from your whole head and face area, don't forget about your tongue, as allowing this to relax in your mouth has a particularly soothing effect.
5. Breathe in and out through your nose as you do all this, saying the word "one" (or any other non-emotive word) silently to yourself each time you finish an inhalation followed by an exhalation.
6. If your thoughts drift, just gently return them to saying your chosen word without forcing anything. It's OK to open your eyes if you need to check the time at any point.
7. When you finish, sit quietly for several minutes, then open your eyes.

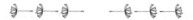

PART II
YOUR REWIND TOOLKIT

Empowering Yourself to Turn Back the Years

"I have chosen to be happy because
it is good for my health."
Voltaire

In this, the largest and arguably most important section of the book, I have divided my insights for you down into thirteen practical chapters (Chapters 6–18) that I hope will serve you well by covering all the main areas that I feel will help you most in your quest to rewind your body clock – from nutrition, gut health, supplements, restorative fasting, herbs, good breathing, vibrant exercise, skin, hair, hormonal balance, the power of relationships and sociability, connecting to nature and restful sleep.

It's up to you whether you choose to work through the chapters in order or to dip in and out of them based on the ones that resonate most with you. Either way, I hope you find the information and exercises on each topic both useful and inspiring – and that on implementing your chosen guidance in your everyday life you will soon start to both *feel* and *see* a difference in terms of overall wellbeing, energy and vitality levels.

Don't forget to read the positive Mindset Phrase at the start of each chapter several times before reading on – whether silently in your own head or out loud – to get you in a frame of mind where you can gain the most from the content that follows. And I hope you also have fun creating your own, personalized Mindset Phrases at the end of each chapter, to help spur you on in your Rewind Journey. Remember: you have more power over how well you age than you think, so dive in and enjoy!

CHAPTER 6

NATURAL NUTRITION

*** I actively choose to feed my body, mind and spirit with nourishment
that lifts me up and moves me toward ever-improving,
abundant health and happiness. ***

Nutrition is a vast topic so, as much as I would dearly love to tell you absolutely all there is to know about anti-ageing nutrition, it would be just too much information and could take up a whole other book! In this chapter I therefore aim to tell you the fundamentals of what you need to know in order to really make a huge difference to your overall wellbeing and rewind your biological age.

I have divided the topics that come under the vast umbrella of nutrition into sections that I hope will make for easier navigation, depending on what you're looking for, so feel free to dip in and out of this chapter any time you want, returning to it time and again. Ultimately, my hope is that the information will enthuse and inspire you to take control of your own nutrition – and maybe even encourage you to help friends and family too.

Weight Loss

First let's address a question that I am constantly asked: "Will following the nutritional advice in this book help me lose weight?"

It is a totally legitimate question and the answer is an honest "YES" if you are carrying extra weight. Conversely, if you are underweight and this is compromising your health, then my recommendations will help you to reach a healthier weight. After all, what we are aiming for here is a sustainable life transformation.

While this is not just a quick-fix "lose 20lbs in a week"-type of book (and we all know those don't work!), the guidance, if followed, will help you become both fitter and leaner for a long, healthy lifetime of looking, feeling and being fantastic. So let's start by looking at the biggest gain of overhauling our diet – reducing inflammation and therefore the risk of the chronic diseases often associated with ageing.

Eating to Reduce Inflammation

An anti-inflammatory diet can actively halt and even reverse biological ageing (see also Chapter 3 on inflammation). There are quite a few approaches out there that claim to be effective, and I have trawled through them, as well as through the mountains of scientific research (and the patient data that I have collected over the past 30 years), so that I can be sure I'm bringing you an approach that is proven to really work, leaving you feeling younger, happier, leaner, brainer and sexier.

The evidence overwhelmingly points to a plant-based, wholefood diet as the best means of reducing chronic inflammation – thus reducing susceptibility to premature ageing. By "plant-based", I'm sure you know that I mean foods that neither contain or are derived from animals (see pages 79–81 for more information); and by "wholefood" I mean food that has been processed or refined as little as possible and is free from additives and other artificial substances.

This information comes from many sources, including the huge Adventist Health Studies (AHS 1 & 2), which began back in the 1960s and looked at the health of over 96,000 people; Seventh-Day Adventists were chosen for this study as they live generally healthy lifestyles and the majority are vegan or vegetarian. The data from these studies show conclusively that these people lived longer, were healthier and were largely protected from diseases of chronic inflammation. And this information is supported by many other large-scale studies, including *The China Study* by Dr T Colin Campbell and his son, which looked at the diets of people living in China and found a correlation between increased meat and dairy consumption and the development of the diseases of ageing.

Essentially a book about one of the biggest scientific research studies ever undertaken, *The China Study* is completely fascinating – I highly recommend it. The study itself has been criticized (not very convincingly) in some quarters, so Dr Campbell revisited it, clarified some of the elements that were refuted and published even more compelling data in a new book called *Whole*. Among the many other proponents of a plant-based, wholefood, vegan diet are the globally renowned and highly respected doctors Frank Sabatino, Caldwell Esselstyn, Michael Klaper, Joel Fuhrman, Neal Barnard and Dean Ornish. In addition, the *British Medical Journal*, Harvard Medical School and the globally respected medical journal *The Lancet* have all gone on record in saying that the healthiest diet, long-term, is a plant-based, wholefood one. So it really is worth thinking about making this dietary change in your own life as part of your Rewind Journey, or at least start taking steps in this direction by beginning to reduce your intake of all meat, dairy and processed foods.

Anti-Inflammatory Cool Foods

In my practice, I see a lot of people with chronic inflammation dramatically helped by introducing cooling foods, such as salads, raw fruit and veg, and dishes cooked at relatively low temperatures, into their diets.

There are many reasons for the anti-inflammatory effect of cool, or cool-producing, foods. It's not that they reduce inflammation because of their cold temperature, as, obviously, whatever we take into our bodies will warm up to body temperature as soon as we swallow it. The therapeutic effects instead happen as a result of these foods being rich in healing and calming phytochemicals that bring us into better balance. Plus, they are hydrating, as they tend to hold more fluid, weight for weight, compared to roasted, grilled or otherwise heated foods. And, last but not least, they have a high vitamin and mineral content, which aids all our systems in healing.

When we cook foods at high temperatures, they have increased levels of Advanced Glycation End-Products (AGEs), which, as we know from Chapter 2, stimulate cells to produce inflammation. While we naturally produce AGEs at a slow rate *ourselves* (endogenous AGEs), consuming food heated to high temperatures means we are taking in a high amount of AGEs from *external* sources (exogenous AGEs) too, which can be very harmful indeed. A Mount Sinai study in 2009 demonstrated lower levels of AGEs in people who consumed foods cooked at lower temperatures compared to people who ate the same foods cooked at higher temperatures.

It has been shown that barbecuing food is even worse for us than just cooking food at high temperatures. This is because grilling foods at a high heat in this way causes charring, which produces potential cancer-causing compounds called heterocyclic amines (HCAs). So if this concerns you as much as it does me, I'd advise steering clear of barbecued food, especially as barbecue *smoke* can also be dangerous – as the food cooks, drops of fat fall and hit the charcoal below, creating toxic chemicals called

PAHs (polycyclic aromatic hydrocarbons) that can damage your lungs. The smoky smell that develops on your clothes, in your hair, and in the environment around the barbecue, is also coating the inside of your lungs. So if you do decide to have a barbecue, the less you can get it to smoke, the less PAH is generated and the less harmful it is.

Now that you have a little insight into a couple of the key components of an anti-inflammatory diet, let's look at the importance of acidity and alkalinity in your diet.

Acid/Alkaline Diets

There are numerous myths these days around the concept of "alkalizing" your body. It seems that we are constantly bombarded with dramatic messages telling us to alkalize. Yet the next moment you'll hear that you can't alter the pH of the body, so there's absolutely no point in trying to "eat alkaline" or to "alkalize".

So, what's the truth? First, let's look at exactly what pH is and why it's important to health. pH is short for "power" or "potential" of hydrogen and is a measure of the acidity and alkalinity of a solution expressed as a number on a scale, where:

- A value of 7 represents neutrality
- Numbers lower than 7 indicate increasing acidity
- Numbers higher than 7 indicate increasing alkalinity
- Each unit of change represents a tenfold change in acidity or alkalinity
- In order to be at our healthiest, our bodies need to maintain a pH of 7.365 (and our body has a low tolerance for variation from this pH)

There's a lot of misinformation around the idea of alkalizing. You may even see claims that "cancer cannot survive in an alkaline environment", which is touted as just one of the reasons to try to make our bodies more alkaline. But this is a misunderstanding as, while cancer cells are indeed found in more acidic environments than healthy cells, this is not because they particularly thrive in an acidic environment but rather because they produce more lactic acid as part of their metabolic process and they therefore *create* a more acidic environment.

Having said this, there is still a compelling reason to try to eat as much alkalizing food as possible, by which I mean mainly fruits, vegetables, legumes and nuts, and to avoid foods considered as acidic – mainly meat, poultry, fish, dairy, eggs, grains and alcohol.

The aim of an alkaline diet is not to try to raise the pH of your blood, per se, but to prevent your body from having to undergo the stress of trying to maintain the healthy pH balance at which it functions optimally.

While we humans evolved with a small acid buffering system, which can easily neutralize the acid caused by our body's *internal* processes (metabolic acids), it's much harder for it to deal with acids taken into the system by consuming acid-forming *foods*, as your body needs to buffer this acid using minerals that we would normally use to keep our bodies healthy. For example, when we are overly acidic, calcium is drawn from our bones and magnesium from our muscles in an attempt to balance our pH, which can lead to many problems including fatigue, mental fuzziness, insomnia, restless leg syndrome and osteoporosis. Interestingly, the naturally alkalizing nutritional recommendations in this book have dramatically helped my fibromyalgia patients – in most cases drastically reducing their pain and discomfort within weeks.

REWIND PRACTICE – OVER TO YOU
Take Your Morning Lemon

Try drinking a glass of lemon water before you do anything else in the morning in order to help maintain an acid–alkaline balance in your body.

Squeeze half a lemon into a glass of warm water and, if you're feeling brave, add a pinch of cayenne pepper – it's an acquired taste, but cayenne is a traditional spice with many health-promoting effects.

It's advised to wait an hour after drinking this mixture before brushing your teeth, though, as acid in foods and drinks can soften your tooth enamel.

Many people erroneously believe that the citric acid in the lemon juice somehow "magically" interacts with the hydrochloric acid in your stomach to become alkaline once you drink it. But the real reason for lemon being alkalizing is that, while it has very high levels of citric acid, it also has very high levels of alkalizing minerals such as magnesium, potassium and sodium, which help to keep your pH level more balanced.

People often ask me why the same trick doesn't work with oranges. The answer is that the sugar content of oranges is so high that it cancels out the benefit of the alkalizing minerals and so has an acidifying effect on the body. Oranges have a wealth of other health-promoting benefits though.

Foods to Help Balance Your pH

It is good to consume plenty of the following foods to support your body in maintaining its pH at the ideal level of 7.365:

- Fruits such as lemons, bananas and cherries
- Dark green, leafy vegetables such as kale, broccoli and beetroot top – both raw and cooked (although avoid eating these raw if you have issues with oxalic acid or hypothyroidism)
- Beans and pulses (for protein)
- Nuts (in moderation due to their high fat content)

Go Organic

Organic eating – by which I mean eating foods produced without the use of chemical fertilizers, pesticides or other artificial chemicals – could easily seem like just a current fad. But when you stop and think about it, it's actually *non*-organic foods that are the *recent* development, given our forefathers lived on a completely organic diet.

Modern farming methods involve the use of genetically modified organisms (GMOs), synthetic fertilizers, pesticides and herbicides, none of which existed in years gone by. And while farming practices and our diet have both been significantly altered over the past century, our bodies and genetics have not, in that it's just not possible to achieve vibrant health when eating a diet that is adulterated with toxic chemicals that your body doesn't recognize and cannot process.

It's therefore advisable to search out food that has not been treated with:

- Pesticides – used to destroy insects or other organisms harmful to the plants being grown
- Herbicides – used to destroy unwanted vegetation
- Ionising radiation – used to improve food safety, shelf life and the like
- Growth hormones – used in factory farming to make animals increase their "yield"
- Antibiotics – used to maintain health in livestock
- Fertilizers from synthetic ingredients or sewage sludge – used to enhance growth

Things like pesticides, herbicides and ionizing radiation are, by their very nature, designed to be toxic to life, so it's not difficult to see why they can be toxic to us too, especially when many of them are fat-soluble. This means that instead of being passed out of your body via your urine, they are stored in your body's fatty tissue and build up there. Eating organic foods will therefore actively help to reduce toxic agro-chemical build-up.

In fact, a study in 2005 demonstrated that, in as little as 15 days, children who adopted a predominantly organic diet experienced a marked decrease in urinary concentrations of organophosphate pesticides. Studies also show that exposure to common food contaminants such as pesticides can seriously affect women's ability to conceive; women who ate more than two daily servings of the 14 fruits and vegetables with the highest pesticide residues (see page 76) were 26 per cent less likely to have a successful pregnancy, compared to women who ate less than one daily serving.

If we choose to eat a lot of meat, fish and dairy, the presence of growth hormones can cause profound disruption to the endocrine system – the body system that produces hormones that regulate metabolism, growth and development, tissue function, sexual function, reproduction, sleep, and mood, among other things.

The overuse of antibiotics in farming is also very worrying as it is resulting in the rapid rise of antibiotic-resistant strains of pathogens, which is, in turn, causing a resurgence of diseases that were previously thought to be virtually eradicated, including deadly tuberculosis. It is estimated that antibiotics may cease to work for medical purposes within as little as the next 10 years due to all the antibiotic-resistant pathogens emerging.

So, if you've been eating a conventional diet for years, now might be a good time to start to cleanse your body of toxic residues by substituting as much of your diet as you can with organic foods.

The Benefits of Going Organic

Many people question the nutritional benefit of organic crops over conventionally grown crops: Are they really worth it – or is it all hype to sell more expensive foods?

A recent study shed new light on the debate, providing evidence that organic foods are richer in nutrients and antioxidants, and lower in pesticides and heavy metals (particularly cadmium).

Other studies suggest that organic soil management increases the production of cancer-fighting compounds called flavonoids in foods, while conventional farming practices involving pesticides, herbicides etc. disturb flavonoid development.

Overall, then, organic crops are not only more nutritious; they also won't deplete your health by putting unwanted and unnecessary toxins in your body.

Getting Started

I know it may seem a little daunting – and expensive! – at first to eat 100 per cent organic. If that's the case, I recommend starting with one food at a time, gradually adding more until you feel ready to make the full switch.

The "Dirty Dozen" and the "Clean 15" are, respectively – as their names suggest – a round-up of the dirtiest, or most chemically contaminated, fruits and veggies, followed by a list of the cleanest, least contaminated ones. These lists tend to change quite often, so it is handy to periodically check for the most up-to-date lists online if you'd like to use them as a guideline for which foods to prioritize going organic with first.

And if you are unable to source any organic foods for whatever reason, then at least ensure that you first wash all foods very thoroughly and then peel them (if relevant) before eating them.

The "Dirty Dozen" and Beyond

Below are the top 12 fruits and veggies that I recommend you prioritise buying in organic form due to the high levels of contamination involved in their standard growing processes:

- Apples
- Blueberries
- Celery
- Cucumbers
- Grapes
- Nectarines
- Peaches
- Potatoes
- Spinach
- Strawberries (currently the most highly contaminated crop, with recent samples showing that strawberries have been exposed to over 25 harmful chemicals)
- Sweet bell peppers
- Tomatoes

Beans and kale are also moving onto this list.

The "Clean 15"

And here follows the 15 "good guys" that you might initially choose to buy in non-organic form given they are not sprayed as heavily with pesticides and have thick skins or peel that cannot be penetrated by chemicals:

- Asparagus
- Avocadoes
- Cabbage
- Cauliflower
- Aubergine (eggplant)
- Grapefruits
- Honeydew melons
- Kiwis
- Mangoes
- Onions
- Peas
- Pineapple
- Sweetcorn (watch for GMOs)
- Sweet potatoes
- Watermelon

Genetically Modified Foods
The following foods are most commonly genetically modified, so should be avoided when possible:

- Alfalfa
- Canola (as in canola oil)
- Corn (including high fructose corn syrup, corn oil, corn syrup)
- Courgette (zucchini) and yellow squash
- Papaya
- Soy (although organic soy is usually not genetically modified)
- Sugar beets (most sugar in Europe is made from this)

Alcohol: Should or Shouldn't We?
One of the most frequent questions I am asked is whether alcohol is bad for you. Although it has long been thought that a small glass of wine a day may help heart disease and a range of other conditions, this is a controversial hypothesis and there are numerous studies that contradict it. There may be value in drinking red wine as it contains a small amount of resveratrol – a powerful antioxidant that is beneficial to a whole range of body systems and processes, that has been shown to possess anti-ageing benefits and that is currently being researched as a Caloric Restriction Mimetic (CRM) (see overleaf).

On the whole, however, I'm afraid alcohol consumption has been shown to accelerate the ageing process despite headlines in the popular media that could be misleading us into thinking otherwise. For example, I recently spotted the following headline gracing the tabloids: "Drinking champagne makes you live longer."

This claim was a bizarre extrapolation from a study conducted on worms! What actually happened was that the researchers discovered that miniscule amounts of alcohol could more than double the lifespan of a tiny worm that scientists frequently use in ageing studies. The amount of alcohol used in the study was 1:20,000, which is roughly equivalent to one small beer being diluted in 100 gallons of water. The UCLA scientists who undertook the study said that the anti-ageing effect could have implications for human health, as we share about 50 per cent of our genes with these worms. Interestingly, however, when the worms were given larger doses of alcohol, it proved to be harmful for them, so the headline didn't quite tell the whole story!

Caloric Restriction

Caloric restriction (CR) is an approach whereby the overall intake of calories is reduced but the overall intake of high nutritional value foods is increased. Think of it as a "Calorie Poor–Nutrient Rich" (CPNR) diet.

Anti-ageing research has really been in full swing since the 1930s, when it was discovered that this caloric-restriction approach dramatically increased not only the lifespan of the animals being studied, but also profoundly improved their health. And since then, when the research was on mice and fruit flies, we now have evidence that CPNR eating benefits the higher primates too, including humans. See pages 108–9 in Chapter 9 for more information on caloric restriction, but for now I'd like to share with you a little about my personal experience of it.

Personal Experience of Caloric Restriction

I have first-hand experience of the dramatic effects of a CPNR diet when I totally changed my lifestyle to combat the serious health problems I mentioned in the Introduction (see page 3). I didn't realize at the time that what I was doing was a CPNR diet. As far as I was concerned, I was just eating super healthily by cutting out all animal proteins, by consuming lots of raw vegetables, fruits, nuts, seeds, sprouted seeds and beans, and by fasting (or feasting) one day a week on green vegetable juices alone. Interestingly, I underwent some tests prior to embarking on this new diet (the ones I mentioned in the Introduction that showed my biological age to be 55 years old). After the first three weeks on my new regime, those biological age tests were repeated, and in that very short space of time my biological age had reduced to 33. And now, after living this lifestyle for the past decade, my biological age measures 25–27 – circa half my chronological age! And, in addition, the devastating health problems from which I suffered for nearly 20 years are under control and I am well, healthy and energetic.

The Benefits of a Plant-Based Diet

One of the reasons a CPNR diet is predominantly, or exclusively, plant-based is that plants provide huge amounts of life-supporting micronutrients, including phytochemicals, vitamins and minerals, with very few exceptions. Plants, when we use them in an unprocessed state, as close to "whole" as we can get, also provide us with all the *macro*nutrients we need: healthy fats, complex carbohydrates – and even proteins! As all these health-supporting goodies happen to be lower calorie, it is easier to get all the nutrients we need without the extra calorie burden of heavily processed foods and animal proteins.

As a plant-based, wholefood diet avoids processed ingredients, focuses on whole foods, uses very little oil, includes virtually no salt and rarely includes added sugars, plant-based eaters tend to have better body composition than people who eat a conventional Western diet.

As a plant-based diet is also low in saturated fat, free of cholesterol, high in fibre, vitamins, minerals and antioxidants, research reveals that following this type of diet will lower your risks of:

- Hypertension (high blood pressure)
- Heart disease
- Diabetes (type 2, and the complications of both types 1 and 2)
- Colon and breast cancers
- Digestive disease
- Obesity

Furthermore, studies show that a plant-based diet can help to reduce body weight and your total LDL (low density lipoprotein) cholesterol levels – often thought of as your "bad cholesterol".

There's a lot of discussion about whether we humans are naturally supposed to be meat-eaters, omnivores or herbivores. Looking at the structure of the human jaw and our intestinal tract, it is now safe to say that we certainly aren't meant to be exclusively carnivorous: we can cope with eating flesh, if necessary, but it's not ideal for us.

Even a quick study of the structure and function of our intestines shows that they are very long in comparison to those of carnivores, and our digestive transit takes much longer too – so animal flesh rots and becomes putrid when travelling though our guts. We therefore do better overall by eating plants, and so does our planet, given that intensive farming practices are destroying our ecology.

Thankfully, more and more people are now coming to an understanding that we do not need to consume animal products in order to get the protein we need. Think of the biggest, strongest animals on the planet – gorillas, elephants, rhinos and even our biggest mammal, the blue whale – all of them live exclusively on plants!

Making the Change to a Plant-Based Diet

The ideal Calorie-Poor, Nutrient-Rich diet is a plant-based, wholefood (PBWF) way of eating that focuses on whole grains, fruits, vegetables, legumes, nuts and seeds and eliminates all animal products, including meat, poultry, fish, eggs and dairy products, such as milk, yogurt, cheese and ice cream, which many of us have been led to believe are good for us.

However, saying goodbye to all these things can be easier said than done. And while a plant-based diet can be a varied, nutritious and delicious way of eating (contrary to what many people believe), making the switch means that you have to initially plan quite a bit more to ensure that all your nutritional requirements are being properly met.

It's important to make sure that you get sufficient protein if you go plant-based, so be sure to incorporate at least some of the following protein-packed foods into your daily diet, allowing for any sensitivities or allergies as always:

- Beans, lentils and split peas
- Quinoa
- Organic soy products, such as tempeh, tofu, soybeans and soy milk
- Nuts and seeds

It's also important to make sure that you get sufficient vitamins and minerals, because healthy bones rely upon adequate supplies of calcium, vitamin D and magnesium, so be sure to:

- Eat plenty of dark green, leafy veggies and beans; both contain calcium.

- Drink plant milks, including soy, almond, rice or hemp milk; these contain both calcium and vitamin D (needed to absorb the calcium).
- Eat mushrooms and fortified cereals, which contain vitamin D. If you aren't consuming fortified foods on a consistent basis, take a vitamin D3 supplement.
- Get out into the sunlight as often as possible or take a vitamin D3 supplement.
- Get enough zinc and iron by eating whole grains, beans and fortified cereals.
- Eat soy products and nutritional yeast for vitamin B12. (See Chapter 8 for more information on supplementation.)

If, however, there's anything that you feel disagrees with you then avoid it. It's always vital to listen to what your body is telling you.

At first glance, a plant-based, wholefood diet may seem restrictive. However, in truth, it is a very rewarding way of eating. Just make sure that you include each of the below four food groups at each meal:

- Plant protein
- Fruit
- Vegetables
- Whole grains

Rainbow on a Plate

Finally, take a look at the colour-based lists below and overleaf for inspiration in terms of the many colourful fruit and vegetables that you can include in your meals. When you plan your meals, think about always "putting a rainbow on your plate" so that you get as big an array of nutrients as possible.

Red Foods

- Beets
- Radicchio
- Radishes
- Red berries
- Red onions
- Red bell peppers
- Red potatoes
- Rhubarb
- Tomatoes

Orange and Yellow Foods

- Apricots
- Butternut squash
- Carrots
- Oranges, tangerines, clementines, etc.
- Pumpkin
- Swede (rutabaga)
- Sweetcorn
- Sweet potatoes
- Yellow beets
- Yellow bell peppers
- Yellow potatoes
- Yellow tomatoes
- Yellow winter squash

Green Foods

- Artichokes
- Asparagus
- Broccoli
- Brussels sprouts
- Calabrese (broccoli rabe)
- Celery
- Chinese cabbage
- Courgette (zucchini)
- Cucumber
- Endive
- Fresh herbs
- Green beans
- Green cabbage
- Green onions
- Leafy greens
- Leeks
- Lettuce
- Okra
- Peas
- Rocket (arugula)
- Snow peas
- Spinach
- Sugar snap peas
- Watercress

The only green foods I recommend avoiding are green bell peppers, as these are not ripe and can cause digestive distress in some people.

Blue, Indigo and Violet Foods
- Aubergine (eggplant)
- Black salsify
- Black olives
- Blueberries
- Potatoes (purple fleshed)
- Purple asparagus
- Purple Belgian endive
- Purple cabbage
- Purple carrots
- Purple bell peppers

White and Tan Foods
- Cauliflower
- Garlic
- Ginger
- Jerusalem artichokes
- Jicama
- Kohlrabi
- Mushrooms
- Nuts and beans of all kinds
- Onions
- Parsnips
- White potatoes
- Shallots
- Tofu, tempeh and seitan
- Turnips
- White corn

Vegan or Plant-Based?
At this point, I'd like to answer a question that comes up time and again – about what the difference is between being "vegan" and "plant-based". It really is a valid point and the answer is that, while both diets exclude animal products, veganism is more of a life philosophy that eschews all animal abuse and cruelty, rather than being just a way of eating. Another difference is that it would be entirely possible to eat an incredibly

unhealthy vegan diet – you could stock up on doughnuts, crisps and cola and still be vegan, for example – whereas these things wouldn't be part of a plant-based, wholefood diet as they are too processed.

And another difference is that a plant-based, wholefood-eating person may still use other animal products such as leather – so although they eat plants, they are not *strictly* speaking fully "vegan". I see myself as sitting at the cross-section in this imaginary Venn diagram in that I eat a plant-based whole food diet and live a compassionate vegan lifestyle. But, ultimately, these terms tend to have slightly different meanings for different people.

REWIND PRACTICE – OVER TO YOU
A Step-by-Step Guide to Going Plant-Based

If you're keen to up your nutritional game as part of your Rewind Journey by switching to the healthy, plant-based approach just outlined, below are some guidelines that you might find useful to help you get started:

- Begin by substituting some or all of your milk and dairy products with soy, rice, almond and hemp alternatives. Try some of the many new tasty vegan cheeses on the market. Instead of conventional yoghurts, opt for the delicious coconut or soy ones.
- Once you are comfortable with these changes, slowly start to exchange some or all fish and animal-derived products (chicken, eggs, turkey, beef, pork, veal, lamb, game and fish) with plant proteins. To do this, you'll need to stock up on nuts and seeds, legumes and beans, and, if they interest you, try some of the vegan meat alternatives, such as tofu, veggie burgers, seitan and tempeh. There are lots of recipes online, so do a quick search for inspiration.
- Gradually add plant-rich smoothies to your diet – particularly ones containing green, leafy veggies (I promise you, they taste great!); see the recipes a little further on in this chapter for some ideas.

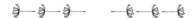

Juices and Smoothies

There is often confusion about the difference between juices and smoothies. They require different equipment to make; their benefits are different; and, in my opinion, it's best to make smoothies on a daily basis, whereas it's best to make juices (ideally vegetable-based juices) when you are doing a detox programme.

Juicing is done in a juicer, with just the juice extracted from the fruit and vegetables, leaving the fibre in the pulp collector at the back of the machine. There are two kinds of juicers most commonly available: centrifugal and masticating. The main appeal of juicing is that it enables you to get a high concentration of nutrients into your body without having to eat huge amounts of fruit and vegetables. This allows your digestive system to rest so that energy can be used for more generalized healing. As you enjoy your delicious juices and absorb various micro- and macronutrients, your body doesn't have to work hard and digest any fibre, so the nourishment is assimilated in a very short amount of time.

Smoothies, on the other hand, are made by blending fruit and vegetables into a thick drink using the whole vegetable or piece of fruit along with plant-based milk or water. The fibre in the raw ingredients remains in the smoothie, which leaves you feeling full and nourished and also ensures regular bowel movements.

A general rule is that it's best to include as many vegetables as possible in both juices and smoothies for the healthiest result, given that vegetables tend to be lower in sugar than fruit and are therefore easier for your body to process in terms of nutrient content. While vegetable juice will keep your blood sugar quite stable, the sugars in fruits go straight into your blood stream, which can cause an unhealthy sugar spike.

You can make smoothies with different combinations of green, leafy vegetables (such as spinach, kale and Swiss chard), with soft fruit such as mango, pineapple and berries, and with superfoods to boost your nutritional intake, such as chia seeds, shelled hemp seed, maca powder, açaí powder, spirulina, chlorella, etc.

Experimentation is key – so have fun coming up with lots of different delicious, health-enhancing concoctions. See both the pages overleaf and my website (JayneyGoddard.org) for inspiration of combinations to try.

Always use organic ingredients wherever possible, particularly if any of the ingredients you use are on the "Dirty Dozen" list (see page 76).

The Joy of Juicing

If I had to tease out one element of my lifestyle that I believe is exceptionally helpful, I would have to say vegetable juicing. When we make juice from fresh organic vegetables, we flood every cell with cleansing, detoxifying nutrients. In fact, when you drink a fresh organic juice, you can often feel the change it makes in your body almost immediately, both feeling and looking brighter, fresher and more energetic etc. On a personal note, I have even noticed facial lines disappearing!

While I'm very aware that this is just my individual experience, research has also been done in this field. In fact, a study that came out just a couple of years ago showed just how what we eat has a very rapid and direct effect on both our appearance and our perceived attractiveness! People in the study were asked to eat two pieces of a high beta-carotene food (carrots, sweet potato, butternut squash, apricots, red and orange bell peppers, and any other orange-coloured fruits and veggies) a day. At the end of the two-week study, they actually looked healthier and more attractive to observers.

Here are some top tips for juicing:

• As already mentioned, use organic produce if possible, as the process of juicing concentrates the foods, so while you're getting massive amounts of nutrients, any toxins present in fruit and vegetables used would also be concentrated.

• Drink your juice as soon as it is made to preserve optimal nutrient value. For example, vitamin C only has a "half-life" after 20 minutes, meaning that half the vitamin C in your drink will have disappeared within just 20 minutes of making it.

• Consider designating one day a week as just a juice fasting (or feasting) day, where you only (or mainly) consume freshly made juices and high-quality water. This has the effect of "resting" your digestive system, allowing healing to happen. It also reduces your overall calorie intake, which contributes to helping you slow your biological ageing.

• Watch the documentary *Fat, Sick and Nearly Dead* – it's an incredibly inspirational story about a man who was very ill and who decided to embark on a juicing programme as he'd tried absolutely everything else to combat a severe health problem. It's a beautiful, feel-good film.

REWIND PRACTICE – OVER TO YOU
Try My Favourite Juice Recipes

Juicing is worth trying any time you'd like a nice, fresh pick-me-up but if you can commit to adding fresh juices to your daily diet for 30 days, you will start to notice a profound difference in your energy levels, health and wellbeing. Here are some of my favourite recipes:

Green Ginger "Ale"

1 cucumber
2 celery sticks
1 apple (a green tart apple is best, as it has less sugar than other varieties)
2cm (0.5in) ginger root, peeled
½ lime

Green Beauty

1 cucumber
2 celery sticks
Handful of kale
(This is a simple juice but it is very "green" and a bit of an acquired taste as it contains nothing sweet. More suited, I'd say, to the "experienced juicer".)

Red Devil

1 raw beetroot
2 carrots
½ lemon
2cm (0.5in) ginger root, peeled

Parsley Woohoo!

Handful of parsley
1 tart apple
2 carrots
1 celery stick
(It's best not to drink this one late at night as the parsley in it will keep you awake with ridiculously high levels of energy – in a good way. Woohoo! You have been warned!)

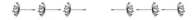

Savouring Smoothies

As already mentioned, smoothies provide massive nutritional bang for your buck! When I teach about the value of smoothies, I always get people to imagine a huge pile of kale on a plate. I ask the audience whether, in all honesty, they would really be able – or willing – to chomp their way through this kale mountain. I've never had anyone say "yes!", yet when the same amount is put into a smoothie, it usually seems entirely manageable. By doing this exercise, I help people to understand that we can get vast amounts of plant nutrition into the body both quickly and easily if we mix it up in a blender. The funny thing is that when you add leafy veggies to a smoothie, you can barely taste them – it's kind of like "stealth nutrition".

REWIND PRACTICE – OVER TO YOU
Try My Favourite Smoothie Recipes

Here are a couple of my favourite smoothie recipes – detoxifying, alkalizing, anti-inflammatory and anti-ageing, as well as refreshing and delicious. Don't worry if you don't have all the ingredients – just make your own version.

Savoury Smoothie

285ml (8fl oz) filtered water (more if needed)
1 chopped cucumber (wash well and use the skin if organic)
½ chopped leek
2–3 chopped celery stalks
¼ bunch parsley or coriander (cilantro)
1 teaspoon turmeric powder
1 avocado, peeled and pitted
1–2 handfuls of sprouted seeds (alfalfa, broccoli, mixed)
2–3 handfuls of curly kale (or spinach, or any other dark green vegetable)

Optional

1 tablespoon spirulina powder
1 tablespoon chlorella powder
2–3 tablespoons raw hemp seeds (shelled)
Splash of coconut or hemp milk
Handful of pumpkin seeds
1 tablespoon maca powder
1 tablespoon chia seeds
1–2 teaspoons mixed seaweed (sea salad)

Sweet Smoothie

½ pint filtered water (more if needed)
¼ teaspoon cinnamon
1 heaped tablespoon raw cacao powder
1 heaped tablespoon raw hemp seeds (shelled)
Handful of goji berries
1–2 handfuls of blueberries or blackberries (can be frozen)
½ teaspoon organic turmeric powder or 1 fresh turmeric root
2cm (0.5in) ginger root, peeled
Few drops of organic Stevia to sweeten, if required

Optional
3 brazil nuts
1 heaped tablespoon maca powder (can be an acquired taste – build up
    slowly)
½ grapefruit, chopped (to be avoided if on anti-hypertensive medication)
½ tablespoon acerola cherry powder
1 teaspoon açaí powder
1 tablespoon baobab powder
1 tablespoon chia seeds
500ml (17fl oz) coconut water

As I lift heavy weights as part of my anti-ageing strategy (see page 142), I
also add a scoop of protein powder to my smoothies. If you would like to
do the same, look for good-quality products that are clearly marked as being
vegan. Some of the best are also "raw vegan". I constantly research and
experiment with different ones, so keep an eye on JayneyGoddard.org to
see which ones I recommend.

Your Nutrition Mindset Moving Forward:

Now that you've come to the end of this chapter, take a little time
to think about its content and come up with a specific, positive,
present-tense Mindset Phrase of your own for the topic in hand, focusing
on the information that has resonated most with you from the chapter.

CHAPTER 7
GUT HEALTH

❝ I gratefully feed and nurture the 100 trillion friendly bacteria in my gut. I know that by lovingly taking care of them, they take care of me. ❞

When we consider that there are, on average, 37.2 trillion cells that make up the human body, and over 100 trillion bacteria cells that inhabit our guts, we have to ask who is actually running the show, as that's quite some ecosystem! In recent years, researchers have developed a far deeper understanding of the important roles played by the 100 trillion or so bugs that we play host to. And, following decades of working out how to kill bacteria with soap and antibiotics, we are coming round to a more sensitive understanding of the symbiotic relationship we have with them.

We've known for some time that certain bacteria in our environment can cause illness. However, only in recent years has it been discovered that the bacteria we host in our digestive system are vital to our health, as they:

- Help to break down the nutrients in our food;
- Synthesize a range of vitamins (particularly the B family);
- Prime our immune systems so that we can recognize pathological (bacterial, viral, fungal, etc.) "enemies";
- Fight off food poisoning;
- Even produce neurotransmitter chemicals that influence our moods.

People with a wide range of diseases, including neurological conditions such as Parkinson's and Alzheimer's and lifestyle-related conditions such as type 2 diabetes and cardiovascular disease have been proven to often have different gut flora from those of healthy people. In addition, people with autoimmune conditions such as rheumatoid arthritis and multiple sclerosis, IBS and type 1 diabetes also have a gut-bacteria profile that differs from the "norm".

Of course, it can be hard to tell whether any of the differences in people with these conditions are brought about as a *consequence* of the condition, or whether the condition *arises* as a result of the different gut-bacteria profile. What we do know, though, is that if we can get a person's gut-bacteria profile right, it makes a dramatic difference to their health – and that by creating optimal profiles we can go a long way to preventing and treating many of the conditions that are associated with premature ageing.

The Importance of Good Gut Bacteria

Our good bacteria, or healthy "microbiome" as it is known, has now been proven to be connected to virtually every aspect of our wellbeing – physical, mental and emotional. When your good bacteria flourish, they can then get on with the job of vitamin production, hormone regulation, toxin excretion and the creation of healing compounds that keep both your gut and you healthy and functioning properly. Here's some strange but fascinating gut health "food for thought":

- The bacteria in our intestine outnumber our body's cells 10 to 1. In that respect, we could be said to be only 10 per cent human!
- Most foods we eat feed only 10 per cent of our cells, and fermentable fibres and resistant starches feed the other 90 per cent.
- Since the 100 trillion+ bacteria living inside us weigh about 3lbs, it isn't surprising that gut flora influences our health to such a degree.
- Imbalances between healthy and unhealthy bacteria are involved in diseases as wide-ranging as obesity, heart disease, autoimmune disease, diabetes, inflammatory bowel diseases and many cancers.
- When our gut bacteria levels are balanced, there's optimal production of short-chain fatty acids (SCFAs), which provide your colon cells with fuel. One of these, called butyrate, can speed up your metabolism, reduce inflammation and help to prevent "leaky gut syndrome", which promotes food allergies, autoimmune disease and weight gain.
- Due to the gut–brain axis and the way our gut has been shown to produce important neurotransmitters, including gut serotonin, bacterial imbalance is also connected with emotional and cognitive disorders including anxiety, autism and depression.

The Carbohydrate Debate

Another gut-health issue that it's important to discuss is the carbohydrate conundrum, about which there's a lot of confusion these days. Some experts say to avoid them and follow a low-carb ("ketogenic") programme while others recommend that we "carb up". Both sides of the argument can seem equally compelling at first glance. However, my position is that all carbs are not created equal and they are therefore not as evil as they are sometimes made out to be, *if* you are eating the *right* type.

We know that eating simple, processed, refined sugars is seriously bad for us. In fact, it is one of the most devastatingly ageing things we can do as it dramatically promotes the formation of AGEs (see Chapter 2, page 42), which make us age rapidly by causing proteins in our bodies, such as the collagen we need for structure, to stiffen. This causes untold internal damage as it compromises many of our organs' ability to function and can even lead to their failure. AGEs also affect our *skin*, causing it to wrinkle as the collagen here stiffens too, breaking and collapsing. So, on the one hand, processed, refined carbohydrates, such as sugar, sweets/candy, white bread, cakes and white rice, should be avoided.

On the other hand, complex carbohydrates found in their natural state in plant-based whole foods, such as organic, short-grain brown rice, sweet potatoes and quinoa, have huge benefits in that they exist in tandem with beneficial phytochemicals (including vitamins and minerals) that are profoundly health-enhancing. Carbohydrates in their natural "whole" state provide a slow release of energy, which has a much lower impact on our blood sugar, keeping it much more stable. These have what we can think of as a "low glycaemic impact", whereas foods that have been processed and refined release their sugars much faster into our bodies, with a potentially devastating effect on our insulin resistance and blood-sugar levels – and a huge impact on the formation of AGEs.

The Discovery of Resistant Starch

A fascinating group of carbohydrates has recently been discovered that provide us with far greater health benefits than simply giving us energy. These carbohydrates are called the resistant starches (RS) and are currently one of the most intensely researched foods.

Resistant starch, as the name suggests, "resists" digestion and is therefore not digested in the small intestine. Instead, our gut bacteria process it, and this creates beneficial molecules that promote balanced blood sugar and healthy gut flora. Resistant starch has many helpful functions, and one of these is that it is a "prebiotic". Prebiotics are a form of food that our healthy gut bacteria feed on, and when we have an abundance of healthy bacteria, nasty bacteria are crowded out.

Adding Resistant Starch to Your Diet

The inclusion of resistant starch in your diet can:

- Improve your metabolism
- Enhance your gut flora, which can help to promote weight loss
- Improve insulin sensitivity and reduce your blood-sugar levels following meals (it can therefore help to reverse type 2 diabetes if a healthy overall diet and other health-enhancing activities are also implemented)
- Improve your blood fats (triglyceride and cholesterol levels) while also decreasing fat mass
- Provide cardiovascular benefits

For quick and easy ways to add resistant starch into your diet:

- Stick to a plant-based, wholefood diet – particularly try to increase your intake of broccoli, aubergine (eggplant), courgette (zucchini), green beans and asparagus.
- Cook, then cool starches such as white potatoes and white rice before eating (these two foods are the only exception to a "no white carbs" rule!). This process changes normal starch to "resistant starch".
- Mix potato starch – easily and cheaply available online or in health stores – into a glass of water, almond milk, and/or your smoothies. I recommend starting with adding about two dessert spoonfuls to your diet each day – for example, one at breakfast and another before bed.

> **Rewind Insight:** Inulin – a type of fibre that is available in powder form as well as in plant foods, such as raw chicory and dandelion leaves, bananas, Jerusalem artichokes, onions, garlic and leeks – is very interesting from an anti-ageing perspective as it has been shown to help to reduce fat around the middle, which tends to accumulate as we age and can become a health hazard. I've recently been starting to add a scoop of inulin to my daily smoothies and have found that I have, without changing any other aspects of my diet or exercise programme, lost 3cm (1.2in) from my waist in a month. That's a pretty fast result!

As resistant starch alters the bacteria balance in your gut, it can initially cause gas and bloating, known as the "die-off effect". However, as the good bacteria crowd out the bad ones, your system will adjust and this will go away.

REWIND PRACTICE – OVER TO YOU
Two Steps to a Healthy Gut

1. Introduce foods to your daily diet that friendly bacteria like to "eat", such as beans and natural inulin sources (see box on page 94). This will create a friendly environment for healthy bacteria to flourish. Also try to include raw oats, unrefined wheat and barley, jicama and yacon if available.

2. Actively introduce friendly bacteria to your gut by eating and drinking the following foods:
   • Kombucha: Watch out for high sugar content if you buy it ready-made. Otherwise, you can buy a starter kit and make your own.
   • Fermented vegetables: Use small amounts of sauerkraut and kimchi if you enjoy them; they're both fermented with strains of beneficial lactic acid bacteria. As an added bonus, many fermented vegetables have a longer shelf life than fresh ones.
   • Miso: This fermented soybean-based product is rich in probiotics because it's made with a "starter" of "koji" (*Aspergillus oryzae*), which is a safe mould with many beneficial properties.
   • Kefir: This is a form of yoghurt usually made from milk. But if you're trying to avoid dairy (and there are a whole host of reasons as to why you should), you can get coconut-based kefirs – or make your own. You just have to buy a starter kit, which a Google search should lead you to.

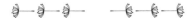

Your Gut Health Mindset Moving Forward:
Now that you've come to the end of this chapter, take a little time to think about its content and come up with a specific, positive, present-tense Mindset Phrase of your own for the topic in hand, focusing on the information that has resonated most with you from the chapter.

CHAPTER 8

SUPER SUPPLEMENTS

" I choose to use only those supplements that are right for me. I carefully select only those natural supplements that I need. "

Vitamins and other nutrients are essential to our wellbeing and how well we age. Ideally, we should get these from our diet – or in the case of vitamin D, from sun exposure. However, due to modern farming methods, there are doubts as to whether it is really possible to get all the micronutrients we need from our food these days for optimal health.

Intensive farming tends to leach minerals in particular from the soil, and over the years important, life-sustaining substances such as selenium, potassium and calcium have therefore become depleted in some areas of the world. "Higher yield" crops also cause problems in that they essentially "dilute" the mineral content, weight for weight. Farmers are taking steps to try to remedy this by adding "supplemented" fertilizers to soil to replace the loss, but this may not always work, so what can we do to help ourselves?

Food vs Supplements

Researchers who were working on a study to find out whether we could benefit as much from taking vitamin supplements as from vitamins in fresh food recently discovered that 100g of fresh apples contained an antioxidant that had vitamin C-like activity equivalent to 1,500mg of vitamin C (about three times the amount of a typical vitamin C supplement). Yet only 5.7mg of *actual* vitamin C was ultimately found in the apples, which is far below the 1,500mg that the level of antioxidant activity associated with vitamin C indicated! In fact, the vitamin C-like

activity from the 100g of apples was an astounding 263 times as potent
as the same amount of the isolated chemical! This is because there are
a huge range of vitamin-C-like compounds in apples, including other
antioxidants such as quercetin, catechin, phlorizin and chlorogenic acid.

Results of studies like this mean that scientists now acknowledge what
qualified complementary medical practitioners have been saying for years:
that whole foods simply give us more nutritional bang for our buck than
any artificial supplementation. This is due to the symphonies of naturally
occurring phytochemicals within them and the profound intricacies of
their interactions with one another as they dance within the food itself –
and then within us as we digest them.

Nutrients obtained from whole foods truly are best for us, but given
that it may not now be possible for us to obtain all the nutrients that we
need from food alone (even if we are lucky enough to have access to the
highest quality fresh food), it is wise for many people to take good-quality
supplements, depending upon each individual's needs.

The Need for Intelligent Supplementation

It goes without saying that vitamin and mineral deficiencies can lead to a
wide range of health issues. Some have been recognized for hundreds of
years, such as scurvy (lack of vitamin C) and rickets (lack of vitamin D)
through to more modern-day problems, including fatigue, anorexia,
obesity, depression and organ malfunction. It is therefore vital to ensure
that you are getting everything you need in order to enjoy optimal health.

To do this, you need to find out your current nutrient status and then,
if it transpires that you are lacking in certain nutrients, you'll need to
know how to intelligently supplement these in your diet. So let's look
at the types of supplement available so that you'll be fully aware of what
to choose, as well as what to avoid, because not all vitamins are created
equal, and the most commonly available ones are actually synthetic.

So what do I mean by a "synthetic" supplement?" Well, I mean
supplements made from chemicals that don't come straight from natural
sources. Under a microscope, they may *look* identical to natural vitamins,
and they may even vaguely *mimic* the way that natural vitamins function
in our body. However, they tend to be what are called "isolates", meaning
that they lack the transporters and co-factors associated with the naturally
occurring vitamins – and therefore cannot be used or recognized by our
body in the same way as the natural version. In their natural form in
plants and other sources, vitamins always appear alongside an array of

other beneficial content, such as phytochemicals, enzymes and minerals, which control the way our body recognizes, metabolizes and uses them to make what it needs. Supplements that replicate this combination of different elements, rather than providing just a vitamin in *isolation*, are therefore called "food state supplements", or "bioavailable supplements", as your body can readily use them.

The Big Deal About Synthetic Vitamins

Unfortunately, more than 95 per cent of all vitamin supplements sold today fall into the synthetic category. And as these isolated synthetic vitamins can't always be used by your body, they are sometimes stored in fat until you obtain the other nutrients required to use them effectively. Alternatively, they are sometimes simply excreted – making very expensive pee!

Another concern is that when synthetic supplements lack necessary trace minerals, they have to use your body's own mineral reserves, which can potentially lead to dangerous mineral deficiencies.

We might not always get what we're expecting from synthetic vitamins and, in fact, we might get a great deal more than we are bargaining for. Just one example of this is the synthetic form of vitamin E. This is referred to as the "dl-" form. The dl-form is a combination of the d-form (which is naturally occurring) and the l-form (which the body doesn't actually use). So it's best to avoid all dl-forms of vitamins by looking out for this on the packaging.

Fat-soluble vitamins (such as A, D, E and K) are especially dangerous in their synthetic forms because a build-up of these in your fatty tissues can cause toxicity. One of the reasons that the synthetic form is more dangerous is that you get a much more highly concentrated serving of the vitamin via the supplement than you would from a food-based form.

Natural or Synthetic?

For a full list of natural versus synthetic supplements, go to my website: JayneyGoddard.org. However, please note that these lists change quite regularly, so do check back from time to time to stay updated. Meanwhile, overleaf are the most common synthetic vitamins to avoid.

Note: Vitamins can come in lots of different forms, so in the list that follows I have provided firstly the common name and then other names to watch out for as these may be listed instead of the common name. Nobody seems to know why this confusing practice takes place, but it does, so it's just a case of paying close attention to the labels on any products you buy.

- Vitamin A: Retinyl palmitate
- Vitamin B1: Thiamine (thiamine mononitrate, thiamine hydrochloride)
- Vitamin B2: Riboflavin
- Vitamin B5: Pantothenic acid (calcium D-pantothenate)
- Vitamin B6: Pyridoxine (pyridoxine hydrochloride)
- Vitamin B12: Cobalamin
- Vitamin C: Ascorbic acid
- Vitamin D: Irradiated ergosterol, calciferol
- Vitamin E: dl-alpha tocopherol, dl-alpha tocopherol acetate or succinate
- Biotin: d-Biotin
- Choline: Choline chloride, choline bitartrate
- Folic acid: Pteroylglutamic acid
- PABA: Para-aminobenzoic acid

And remember: the dl- form of any vitamin is synthetic. Other toxic ingredients to avoid in supplements include:

- Carnauba wax (which is used in car wax and shoe polish)
- Magnesium stearate (or stearic acid)
- Monosodium glutamate (MSG; often disguised as "natural flavours")
- Titanium dioxide (which is a carcinogen)
- Dicalcium phosphate (inorganic calcium that may provoke side effects including kidney stones, diarrhoea and vomiting)
- Cellulose
- Crospovidone (which is related to formaldehyde; manufacturers claim it is inert but it has been found in people's lungs post-autopsy)

REWIND PRACTICE – OVER TO YOU
Find Out What Supplements You Need

I strongly suggest that if you're interested in taking supplements to help in your quest for longevity, you ask your doctor or complementary health professional to get you tested for what you actually need rather than taking a scatter-gun, best-guess approach.

There is a chance that anyone who follows a plant-based diet (or even an animal-protein-based diet) may, for example, lack vitamin B12, occasionally D3 and the essential fatty acid omega 3 (which is best to get as an extract from algae rather than as a fish oil. It is called "vegan omega 3 – algal form"). And, happily, healthy levels of all of these are very easy to maintain with vegan supplements if required.

I always get my patients tested so that I can be sure there is a valid health reason for recommending any supplement to them. You'll find an array of tests that you might like to consider on my website: JayneyGoddard.org.

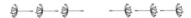

Your Supplement Mindset Moving Forward:
Now that you've come to the end of this chapter, take a little time to think about its content and come up with a specific, positive, present-tense Mindset Phrase of your own for the topic in hand, focusing on the information that has resonated most with you from the chapter.

CHAPTER 9
RESTORATIVE FASTING

❝ I gently rewind my body clock by taking occasional rests from food. I choose to fast only when I need to and know that it will be beneficial for me. ❞

One of the most powerful techniques we can use to get biologically younger – and to address some of the most profoundly debilitating health conditions – is to introduce fasting into our lives. However, fasting is a much-misunderstood topic, so, in this chapter, we'll explore a number of approaches to it, complete with the benefits and pitfalls of each, so that you have the facts before taking any action. You'll firstly find out about the incredible power of water-only fasting, then you'll hear more about caloric restriction (not *strictly* speaking a form of fasting but included here as some people conflate it with this and it's interesting to consider), and finally you'll read about the different types of intermittent fasting.

Water-Only Fasting
I first discovered just how powerful fasting can be when I was experiencing a major flare-up of my rheumatoid arthritis in 2014. I had been in remission for quite a while and was virtually symptom-free. However, typically for me back then, I had been overworking and not taking care of myself as well as I should have been. The irony was that I was putting together my first major health retreat. As a result, I was burning the candle at both ends and getting very tired and anxious. So, it was no surprise that my symptoms came back with a vengeance. I had a blood test and my CRP (a marker of inflammation) level was extremely high at 45 – it

should ideally be less than 3. My body was mounting an all-out attack on itself. But I really wanted to run the retreat as I knew it was fantastic and would help so many people, so failure just didn't feel like an option to me. I needed to do something – and quickly – to get back on track.

I had previously met Dr Frank Sabatino, DC, PhD, one of the world's leading water-only fasting doctors, and explained my situation, and he had recommended a seven-day water-only fast, kindly agreeing to supervise me. As the name suggests, a water-only fast is where you only drink water and take no food whatsoever. My first response to this was one of fear. How would I survive on water alone for a whole week? Would I be able to cope with being so hungry? Is it dangerous? Would it work? Dr Sabatino kindly explained that all these responses were normal as we are all so conditioned to eat that the idea of going without food tends to feel pretty alarming. And it turns out that water-only fasting is a curative that has been used for centuries and is totally safe if you are a suitable candidate for it and you are properly supervised (see pages 104–5 for guidelines and contraindications).

So I embarked on my first supervised water-only fast, and yes, it was quite hard-going for the first day, but I'd mentally committed to seeing it through, so I just went with the process – and by the second day I was feeling OK and didn't even feel hungry!

It's vital to rest when fasting, so I did. I gathered the books I'd been intending to read for ages and dipped into them between resting. The really intriguing thing was that my body just seemed to know what to do – a bit like the way in which a sick animal will hide away and do nothing but rest until it is better. And I was surprised that I slept really well at night – despite the on-and-off snoozing throughout the day.

Now, I happened to have a blood test booked to check my CRP levels on the fourth day of the fast, so, although I should have been resting, I went along anyway as I was curious to find out whether the fast had had any effect on my inflammation. I got the results of the test the next day and found out that my CRP had dropped from 45 right down to 2! Pretty amazing after just four days of fasting!

The process known as "refeeding" is another of the most important parts of a water-only fast and must be carefully monitored by a trained supervisor. I finished my supervised fast on Day 7, breaking it with diluted green juice (just cucumber and celery) on Day 8. I then progressed to full-strength juice on Day 9 and 10 before being allowed to have a tiny piece of watermelon in the afternoon of Day 10 – and watermelon has never tasted so good! Next, I was allowed to eat small vegetable-only salads, and finally Dr Sabatino allowed me to go back to my normal, mainly raw, plant-based diet on Day 14.

The Benefits

Doing a water-only fast made a huge difference to my health in every respect. It was like a reset button, and I now periodically do it whenever I feel the need.

Because I fast about four times a year, a three-day fast tends to be enough for me (with a careful three-day refeed) as my system responds quickly. That's just the way my metabolism works; yours may be different.

I feel that water-only fasting is one of the most incredible rapid health-enhancement tools available. It is so elegant in its simplicity yet so profoundly effective. Following my fast and refeed, I looked and felt better than ever. People kept remarking on my "glow", and my energy levels were very high. And, as for that retreat? Well, I'm happy to say that it was an outstanding success – and had I not fasted, the outcome is likely to have been very different.

Some Guidelines

While fasting has been used therapeutically for millennia, it is only now being incorporated in conventional medicine. Below are some crucial guidelines to follow to ensure that it is safe for you:

- Never attempt a water-only fast for longer than three days without expert supervision.
- Correct advance preparation is essential for fasting: it's advised that you transition to a plant-based, wholefood diet if you don't already eat that way, and make your meals more salad- and fruit-based for about a week or longer before a fast as you'll experience less "detox" discomfort.
- Take complete bed rest and psychological rest while fasting – so no working or stressing.
- Gradual refeeding after fasting is essential, as per the example I explained opposite.

Contraindications

Also, crucially, do NOT water-only fast if you have, or are affected by, any of the below conditions. Note that this list of contraindications is not definitive, and as new research comes to light, conditions may be added to or removed from the official list, so please do check on a reputable website or liaise with a professional before embarking on a fast:

- Drug therapy causing protein wasting (steroids, antineoplastic agents)
- Major system failure (liver failure, renal failure)
- Malignant arrhythmias
- Metastatic cancers
- Pregnancy or lactation
- Protein wasting disease (lupus, Cushing's syndrome)
- Unstable angina

It also important to approach fasting with caution if you have, or are affected by, any of the following:

- Angina or a history of heart disease
- Chronic drug therapy (insulin, oral hypoglycaemics, anti-inflammatory agents, psychotropic agents)
- Congestive heart failure
- Drug therapy with potassium-wasting diuretics, adrenergic stimulating agents
- History of failure of compliance with medical regimens
- History of kidney or gallbladder stones or suspected kidney or gallbladder stones, as water fasting – and perhaps even juice feasting – can catalyse the elimination of stones which can be very painful
- History of psychiatric or emotional disorder
- Presence of systemic disease
- Rapid heartbeat (supraventricular tachycardia)
- Substance abuse

How Water-Only Fasting Works

The truly therapeutic part of a water fast does not actually begin until the second or third day. The reason for this is that during the first 24–48 hours, your body is still burning off circulating blood sugar as well as sugar stored in the muscles and liver in the form of glycogen.

Once the first two to three days of the fast are over, your body then begins to burn fat tissue for fuel. Next, molecules called ketones begin circulating in the blood. These suppress hunger, which is why fasting is not as difficult as you might think once you are over the first few days.

Many people don't understand the process of ketosis correctly (when the body is in a metabolic state in which some of the body's energy supply is coming from ketones in the blood, rather than from the normal blood glucose). There is therefore sometimes a fear that it could lead to loss of consciousness or even more dire consequences. However, a respected group of hygienic physicians (as doctors working in this field are known) have supervised many thousands of water fasts over many years, and have shown these concerns to be unfounded. In fact, when fasting is undertaken in a supportive environment, with the supervising practitioner ensuring proper hydration and total resting conditions, kidney and heart function often dramatically improve as weight and blood pressure drop. As a result, there is often a great improvement in the acuity of the senses; vision, hearing, touch, taste and sense of smell.

Dr Sabatino explains that the adjustment the brain makes to ensure its stability via ketones in the absence of food intake is a unique one, as brain cells are one of two directly glucose-dependent cells of the body. Since the brain is responsible for running all our cognitive and biological functions, it makes its energy needs top priority.

An interesting observation is that when brain cells become cancerous, they lose the ability to utilize ketones for energy. This means that if someone with brain cancer was put on a sugar-free diet, or even more powerfully, water-only fasting, cancer cells and tumours in the brain could potentially be starved, shrunk and destroyed to some degree.

REWIND PRACTICE – OVER TO YOU
Get Into the "Benefit Mindset" for Fasting

The idea of going without food for even a relatively short time is, for many, an initially daunting prospect. However, instead of thinking about everything that you are missing, try to positively re-frame the process in terms of the benefits that will come your way if you go for it!

A study by researchers at the University of Southern California found thatrefraining from food for as little as two days can regenerate the immune system. Isn't that incredible! And fasting for two to four days helps the body to fight infection as well as flipping "a regenerative switch" that triggers stem-cell-based regeneration of new white blood cells, thereby renewing the body's entire defence system.

Essentially, then, during a fast, the human body is able to get rid of the parts of the immune system that are either damaged, inefficient or simply old! So what is there not to like about *that*?

Caloric Restriction: Living Longer by Eating Less?

We already touched on the topic of caloric restriction – or "CR" as it is known to aficionados – as an important anti-ageing and potential life extension tool in Chapter 6, "Natural Nutrition" (see pages 69–89). However, we're going to look at it again here even though, as I mentioned at the start of this chapter, it's not *strictly* speaking a form of fasting as *such*.

CR is very different from a low-calorie diet, the primary aim of which is usually to lose weight. As explained on page 78, it is instead an approach whereby, as the name suggests, you eat fewer calories, but the overall intake of *high nutritional value* foods and drinks is increased. In order to reap the full anti-ageing benefits that CR can bestow, you'd need to reduce your overall calorie intake by about one quarter to one third.

Traditional CR programmes – where people eat a standard omnivorous diet but just a lot less of it – would be a huge challenge for most people, requiring them to take great care that a full array of vitamins, minerals and other necessary dietary elements were present in their amended diet.

I met some dedicated traditional "CR lifestylers" at a recent anti-ageing medical conference in the US and they seemed totally preoccupied with the regime, almost treating it as a full-time occupation. They were a very dedicated group of individuals who weighed and measured each morsel of food and drink that they consumed, as well as doing all the hundreds of calculations required to absolutely ensure that they were getting the right amounts of nutrients. And while doing this can yield amazing results in terms of overall health and vitality, not many people are likely to have either the time or inclination to go to such lengths.

If, on the other hand, someone is willing to make the switch to a plant-based, wholefood diet that doesn't have the calorie density of animal-based foods, CR is likely to be easier to achieve given it's a lot easier to fill yourself up without piling on the calories. Most vegans, if eating a wholefood diet, are actually unintentionally participating in a CR regime.

Calorie Restriction Pills?

At present, there aren't any viable alternatives to physically reducing calorie intake by whatever food methods one chooses to use. However, it's worth noting that scientists are working on finding ways that we can eat a "normal" amount of food but trick our bodies into responding as if we are consuming fewer calories by taking substances known as Caloric Restriction Mimetics (CRMs). One of the most promising emerging compounds in this area is called resveratrol, which is a naturally occurring substance derived from red grapes and other plant sources – particularly

Japanese knotweed. For anyone who might want to look further into this, it's important to look for the more effective trans-resveratrol (rather than the cis-resveratrol) version of the supplement.

Overall, however, I'm not a fan of CRMs personally as, to me, the danger is that, should these substances genuinely produce the CR effect, it almost gives the message that "you can just eat rubbish, take a pill and all will be fine". This could lead to malnourishment at best and premature ageing and descent into devastating disease at worst.

We humans are still intrinsically drawn to the high-calorie foods that were so important to our energy levels for survival as we evolved. However, we no longer need to walk miles to forage for a few nuts and berries, and we certainly don't have to defend our families against sabre-tooth tigers, so such high-calorie foods really serve no truly *useful* role in our nutritional tapestry any longer. As such, I don't yet see a vibrant, healthy future where we could just pop a CR pill and eat half a dozen doughnuts with impunity! Surely, it must be better to teach ourselves to be more knowledgeable and more disciplined about nutritious food intake, whether we decide to dip our toes into the world of caloric restriction or not, than to mindlessly stuff our faces with lots of convenience and junk food that ultimately serves no function in terms of helping us to maintain healthy, vibrant bodies and minds?

Intermittent Fasting

Another form of caloric restriction that has become popular within recent years in the wellness community – primarily as a way of losing weight but also due to wider health benefits – is known as intermittent fasting (IF).

The most popular IF programs are the 5:2 diet and the 8:16 diet. On 5:2, you eat normally for five days and then reduce your caloric intake for two non-consecutive days of the week. On 8:16, you only eat during an 8-hour window and consume nothing for the remaining 16 hours in a 24-hour period. While people often do lose weight on such programmes, they can't really be considered "fasting" as such, as food is being eaten.

In a fascinating study by Dr Mark Mattson and his team at the USA's National Institute on Ageing, mice were genetically "programmed" to develop Alzheimer's disease in the same way that humans would. These trials demonstrated that the onset of Alzheimer's could be delayed by the equivalent of 30 years in mice fed on an intermittent fasting regime, which translates to postponing the age of onset in humans from 50 to 80 years of age! "Intermittent Energy Restriction" – the correct term for Dr Mattson's protocol – consists of normal feeding and restricted feeding on alternate days. In humans this would equate to eating normally on one day and then eating 400–500 calories for women, or 500–600 calories for men, on fasting days. Dr Mattson claims that the evidence for intermittent fasting working in *humans* is "very good to excellent".

Unfortunately, because we humans love to be entertained, and food does that very well, a lot of the books on intermittent fasting make the promise that you can eat whatever you want as long as you fast on the other days. But, clearly, we know that this is not true. Intermittent fasting gets much better results – from a total wellbeing perspective – if a healthy diet is eaten and other positive lifestyle activities are included, such as exercise, mindfulness, socializing and more. My personal take is therefore that this protocol would be even better if there was more of an emphasis on *healthy* food consumption – ideally a plant-based diet, the benefits of which I've already espoused on pages 79–80.

How to Choose the Right Fasting Path

To reiterate, the water-only fasting discussed on pages 103–7 is the only *genuine* form of fasting; the other two approaches included in this chapter are simply effective methods of caloric restriction.

Water-only fasting can be a particularly useful thing to do if you're unwell and in need of drastic change – if your condition doesn't contraindicate this approach, of course – or simply if you're in search of great transformation. However, it is essential that you fast under supervision. One of the best resources to find professionals properly trained and qualified in supervising this type of fast is the Natural Health Association (NHA; www.healthscience.org).

If you'd like to reduce your calorie intake to lose body fat, you might prefer to consider an intermittent fasting (IF) approach, which generally doesn't need supervision. And if you're looking at an overall age-rewind strategy, caloric restriction (CR) around a plant-based, wholefood diet can be a great solution.

Of course, as with all approaches in this book, it's crucial to use your common sense to ensure that your chosen method is safe for you, checking with a health professional if in doubt.

Your Fasting Mindset Moving Forward:

Now that you've come to the end of this chapter, take a little time to think about its content and come up with a specific, positive, present-tense Mindset Phrase of your own for the topic in hand, focusing on the information that has resonated most with you from the chapter.

CHAPTER 10
HERBS FOR YOUTHFUL VITALITY

" I harness the mighty power of herbs for my health and longevity. I respect the potency of these gifts of nature and use them with thoughtful care. "

I'm always fascinated by the way the herbs that we commonly use in our food can double up as powerful medicine – with many of them having a profound effect on age reversal and youth-promotion. Being the wellness geek that I am, I find it impossible to walk down a country lane without making a mental note of all the incredible medicines in the hedgerows that are available to us all – if we just knew how to harness their powers.

In this chapter, I will share with you the herbs and spices that have the most impact when it comes to reversing the cellular damage that accrues as we age, including giving guidance on some rejuvenating potions and lotions that you can make for yourself. I'll also introduce you to the fascinating world of adaptogenic herbs, which are particularly effective in helping to restore us to a state of healthy balance in times of extreme stress.

Herbs for Longevity

You will find overleaf a countdown of the top 12 herbs that I rate, based on scientific evidence, as the most effective in helping us to remain disease-free and biologically younger, each one with a summary of its key benefits.

12. Rosemary: To Enhance Memory and Hair Growth

The old phrase, "rosemary for remembrance", which Shakespeare included in *Hamlet*, has sunk into the common psyche, showing that our ancestors clearly knew that this herb is linked with improving memory. And rosemary is still used today in remembrance posies.

Rosemary is also commonly used in natural products, including supplements, as a preservative due to its powerful antioxidant properties.

Furthermore, in studies, rosemary essential oil has been shown to be extremely helpful in promoting hair growth – even where it has been lost due to excess testosterone (such as in male pattern baldness, a condition that can also affect women if they have hormonal imbalances). Interestingly, rosemary actually performs better than conventional hair growth and restoration topical treatments. See page 173 for guidance on how to make your own rosemary hair restorer.

11. Spearmint: To Calm the Stomach and Boost Energy

This fresh-tasting herb has powerful antioxidant properties and is well known for its ability to help with digestion and calm an upset stomach. It can relieve the symptoms of IBS in some and, from an anti-ageing perspective, research indicates it can be helpful in combatting certain chronic diseases. It has also been shown to help polycystic ovarian syndrome (PCOS) by inhibiting and stimulating the endocrine system in various ways, thus improving hormonal balance and preventing the many metabolic side effects of PCOS, including hirsutism.

Rewind Insight: A study from St Louis University found that extracts from spearmint and rosemary used together can improve learning and memory quite dramatically. I created my own "brain performance" spritz when I was writing my MSc dissertation, and I'm using the same recipe while writing this book. It really helped me both then and now.

To make your own, simply combine a few drops of rosemary and spearmint essential oil with water in a spray bottle (a plant spray bottle would work well) and spritz into the air. This will enable you to retain and recall information more readily, so is particularly useful for anyone studying or suffering from dementia of any kind.

As the iron content of spearmint is high, it can stimulate the production of red blood cells and haemoglobin, thus also helping to prevent anaemia as well as enhancing general circulation, energy levels and wound-healing.

10. Basil: The Spicy Italian Secret for Younger-Looking Skin

Herbs traditionally used in Italian cooking tend to contain high levels of antioxidants, and basil is a particularly good example of this. As such, it protects us from harmful free radicals – the damaging molecules that can lead to degenerative issues including skin wrinkling, osteoporosis, heart disease, many cancers and even neurological diseases such as Alzheimer's.

Basil can be used as a herb in food or in teas, and its essential oil is an extremely powerful antidote to sickness and diarrhoea. It is also an anti-spasmodic, so can help to relieve coughs, and research shows that it may be beneficial for asthma sufferers, too.

Basil essential oil has a refreshing effect, so can also be used to help relieve nervous tension, mental fatigue and feelings of melancholy. It is also a powerful remedy for migraines, promoting mental strength and clarity.

9. Marjoram: For Both Better Digestion and Better Sleep

A good night's sleep is essential to your overall wellbeing (see Chapter 18 for more on this), and research shows that adding marjoram to your diet may well improve digestion, which can lead to better sleep. Another way of benefiting from marjoram's relaxing properties would be to add a couple of drops of the essential oil to a warm bath before going to bed.

Marjoram oil has a pleasant warming effect on your body and improves circulation, which increases blood flow, further warming and nourishing your cells. It can also be used to help clear coughs and excess phlegm, and is effective at relieving the pain of arthritis and rheumatism.

Research shows that marjoram oil also helps to improve cognitive function and suggests that it might therefore be able to help prevent debilitating neurological conditions including Alzheimer's disease and dementia, as it helps to stop the formation of excessive beta-amyloid plaques which are linked with worsening Alzheimer's in particular.

8. Thyme: For Frequent Infections

Frequent infections can really take a toll on our general health, causing us to age biologically. Studies have shown that the humble herb thyme has the power to disable the MRSA bacteria, which could otherwise lead to deadly infections. Essential oil of thyme also makes a very effective mouthwash, which can effectively treat inflammation, gum disease and sore throats. It's also a great addition to an essential oil room spritz as it cleanses the atmosphere. Plus it's ideal for disinfecting rooms where sick people have been as it really knocks germs for six.

7. Sage: To Fight Inflammation

As explored in Chapter 3, inflammation is one of the key underlying causes of premature ageing. Sage is a superb anti-inflammatory and therefore helps to counteract the problems caused by autoimmune diseases such as rheumatoid arthritis and other inflammation-driven conditions such as asthma. The anti-inflammatory qualities of sage also extend to preventing and improving the symptoms of gout, as well as reducing inflammation of the cardiovascular system, thus potentially helping with high blood pressure and heart issues.

Sage is also known to strengthen the immune system, enhance brain function, regulate digestion, strengthen the bones, slow the onset of cognitive disorders, and prevent and assist recovery from type 2 diabetes.

Even small amounts of sage, whether consumed as a herb or inhaled as a diluted oil, can improve memory retention and recall abilities. Brain activity monitoring studies show that it increases capacity for concentration on a chosen topic, so it is ideal for anyone who feels they need to improve their focus for any reason.

Sage has quite an intense flavour, but actually chewing on the leaves is one of the very best ways to get its volatile oils into your system. If, however, that feels like too much for you, then the herb can be used in small quantities to make a tincture or tea instead.

Due to the antimicrobial properties of the herb, it can also be nice to make a sage salve to help prevent bacterial and viral infections that attack the body through the skin. We often think of illness entering through our nose or mouth, but the skin can also be compromised (think cuts, rashes and grazes) and be an entry point for pathogens.

Most people aren't aware that sage also has high levels of vitamin K – an important vitamin that isn't found in many foods. Vitamin K is crucial for maintaining bone density as we age. So if you suffer from osteopenia (early stages of osteoporosis) or have lived a sedentary, nutrient-poor lifestyle, it could be helpful to add sage to your diet to help with bone health.

Sage also contains a variety of chemicals that mimic the drugs typically prescribed for managing type 2 diabetes. As such, it appears to regulate and inhibit the release of stored glucose in the liver, preventing major fluctuations of blood sugar, and either helping to prevent the onset of type 2 diabetes or helping to manage and improve the condition if it has already manifested.

6. Ginger: To Warm the Cockles of Your Heart

Delicious warming ginger has a whole range of amazing healing uses, so you'd best brace yourself for this one.

Its anti-inflammatory properties can help to keep your heart healthy and your arteries clear. It has also been shown to help improve immune system function, to lower cholesterol levels and to help prevent the formation of oxidized LDL ("bad" cholesterol).

Ginger has also been shown to boost metabolism, therefore potentially accelerating weight loss. Interestingly, it also increases exercise endurance capacity, so feel free to try consuming more ginger if you'd like to be able to work out harder and longer.

Organic compounds within ginger – gingerol in particular – have also been extensively studied for their cancer-prevention properties. For example, gingerol is thought by some to be helpful in the prevention of both breast cancer and skin cancer. Furthermore, recent studies have also linked gingerol to healthy cell death (apoptosis) in ovarian cancer cells, and this can help to reduce the incidence of tumours – and the growth of cancerous cells – without harming the healthy cells around them. Another powerful compound in ginger, zerumbone, has been linked to helping with the prevention of gastric, ovarian and pancreatic cancer as it is an anti-angiogenic, which means it could prevent the growth of blood vessels in tumours. As such, it is being researched as a potential anti-tumour drug.

Ginger can also help to balance blood-sugar levels in people suffering from type 2 diabetes. Plus, it is thought to help with the onset of age-related, neurodegenerative diseases such as dementia and Alzheimer's, as it is a potent antioxidant and helps to keep your memory intact.

Finally, I thought you'd also like to know that ginger has been used for years to enhance desire and sexual activity. The root helps increase blood circulation, particularly to the mid-section of the body, which is, of course, an important area for sexual performance.

5. Oregano: To Protect Your Bones and Aid in Detox

Oregano is a nutrient-rich herb, containing high levels of calcium, iron and manganese, and this makes it great for protecting your bones against osteoporosis later in life. The active constituent of oregano, called rosmarinic acid, helps to eliminate free radicals that age us and contribute to disease. The herb also contains organic compounds that make it very useful for supporting your body's detoxification pathways. Plus it contains a form of omega-3 fatty acid that helps to rebalance cholesterol levels and reduce cardiovascular inflammation, enhancing overall health.

4. Allspice: The Caribbean Anti-Ageing Secret

Allspice is a potent spice from Jamaica that has a complex and intriguing mix of flavours. It can help to keep blood-sugar levels under control by balancing circulating blood glucose, which helps to inhibit the formation of AGEs.

If incorporated into a healthy diet, it also helps to improve circulation, enhance mood, protect the gastrointestinal system, enhance healthy immune function, lower blood pressure and reduce chronic inflammation. Plus it has pain-relieving qualities.

Allspice also has antibacterial and antifungal properties and is particularly potent in combatting unhealthy stomach bacteria (*E. coli* and *Listeria monocytogenes*, in particular). When added to foods, it can even deactivate harmful bacteria before they start to do damage.

The presence of a variety of potent chemical compounds, including eugenol, tannins and quercetin, make allspice a potent antioxidant too. And the high levels of vitamins A and C in the spice add to this antioxidant activity.

Allspice is also an effective vasodilator, relaxing blood vessels, allowing increased blood to flow through them, therefore reducing the strain on the heart and arteries and lowering the risk of us developing conditions such as atherosclerosis, strokes and heart attacks.

3. Cloves: Superhero of the Spice World

Cloves beat the other spices so far hands down when it comes to anti-ageing properties as they have the highest antioxidant levels, so regular consumption of cloves is a good idea as part of your Rewind Journey.

Most of us are familiar with clove oil being used, with caution, as an anaesthetic for toothache, gum pain and sore throats. However, cloves can also offer relief from respiratory problems including bronchitis and asthma and they help to fight intestinal parasites, bacterial overgrowth and fungal infections. They have also been shown to aid digestion, protect the liver, improve immune system function, support improved blood sugar metabolism and preserve bone density, as well as being researched as an anti-cancer agent. Last but not least, they have potent aphrodisiac properties, so can help to keep things vibrant on that front, too.

2. Cinnamon: Queen of Anti-Ageing Spices

Cinnamon contains anti-inflammatory compounds that have been shown to help relieve pain. However, one of the most exciting benefits it gives us is its ability to help our bodies deal with sugar better. In fact, just a quarter of a teaspoon of cinnamon a day has been proven to reduce blood--sugar levels. Cinnamon is also a Caloric Restriction Mimetic (CRM; see page 108), which means it has the ability to mimic the effects of a low-calorie diet and therefore slow signs of biological ageing.

Research into cinnamon's effects on cancer has been ongoing for many years, and two substances in particular – cinnamaldehyde and eugenol – have been shown to actively prevent cancer cells spreading and growing, which is an exciting development for cancer research, particularly in the case of colon cancer, lymphoma and leukaemia. These antioxidant constituents are also markedly beneficial for skin health and appearance, and they enhance your body's ability to heal and repair itself.

There is also an intriguing chemical connection between your brain and the scent and taste of cinnamon. So much so that, in research, when people chewed cinnamon-flavoured gum, or simply smelled cinnamon, their cognitive ability was proven to be enhanced!

1. Turmeric: Pure Anti-Ageing Gold!

Turmeric is the spice that gives many curries that beautiful yellow colour. A potent anti-ageing agent, it is loaded with antioxidants, which help to fight the signs of ageing, including reducing wrinkles and lessening hyper-pigmentation from sun damage by curbing the growth of free radicals.

In India, where turmeric is extensively used, the incidence of the four most common cancers found in developed nations is ten times lower. It is thought that this phenomenon is at least in small part due to the regular consumption of turmeric, which contains many active compounds, the most potent of which is curcumin. This is one of the most widely researched spice extracts, and studies strongly suggest that it can help protect us against cancer and can even instigate cell death that is helpful in diminishing tumours while allowing normal cells to function properly (a process called apoptosis). Curcumin has also been shown to help protect against Alzheimer's, coronary artery disease and any condition where chronic inflammation is the underlying cause.

Turmeric's active compounds have also been shown to enhance liver function, which helps to reduce levels of toxicity in the body. And the antioxidant properties of turmeric can be helpful for liver ailments such as cirrhosis and fatty liver disease.

Historically, turmeric has often been used to enhance cognitive abilities, improve concentration and enhance memory retention, and modern-day research has proven that these traditional approaches have validity. It has also been shown to help protect neural pathways from long-term oxidative stress and the build-up of harmful substances.

Note: Remember that, as with all foodstuffs, herbs and spices have the potential to provoke an allergic response in some people. Furthermore, some should be used with caution during pregnancy and breastfeeding. Do check with a qualified herbalist if you are in any doubt whatsoever as to whether a particular herb or spice is safe and/or appropriate for you.

REWIND PRACTICE – OVER TO YOU
Choosing and Using Your Herbs

Now that you have lots of juicy information about what I consider to be the top 12 anti-ageing herbs, consider which ones sound most likely to be beneficial for you on your Rewind Journey, given where you are right now. Then use the list below of different ways to weave the amazing power of herbs into your daily life to decide which approaches you feel would work best for *you*. Make a note of these in a notebook or your journal so that you positively reinforce your decision.

- Include them in salads – this works with any fresh herbs and spices, so choose the ones you like best
- Add them to smoothies – I particularly love adding ginger, turmeric and/or cinnamon; and a pinch of cayenne boosts circulation
- Make a tea with them by picking the leaves of any of the fresh herbs that resonate with you and steeping them in boiling water for several minutes, checking for any allergies or reactions, of course
- Make a salve from them to apply to the skin (see the suggestions and guidance on pages 124–5)

Harnessing the Mighty Power of Adaptogens

In striving for optimal wellbeing and vitality, there's nothing more important than being in a state of balance – not just physically but also mentally and emotionally. All well and good – in theory. However, the fact is that, in the real world, there will always be things that knock us off centre, whether you're running a marathon, dealing with chicken-pox afflicted kids, a rather overly vigilant mother-in-law, pressing work deadlines, rather too many late nights with your latest flame, or family bereavement.

Happily, there are "secret herbal weapons" that we can employ to support ourselves through particularly stressful periods so that the stress just doesn't affect us so much – and which will help us to maintain at least some kind of equilibrium. These are called "adaptogens".

Adaptogenic herbs have a long history of use throughout healing traditions all over the world. In ancient (and also not so ancient) times, they were considered to be tonics or rejuvenators, and would have been prescribed, prepared and dispensed by the community's wise woman. In 1947, pharmacologist and toxicologist Dr Nikolai Lazarev coined the term "adaptogen" to specifically describe a plant that helps one to "adapt" to stressful circumstances – physically, mentally or emotionally. For a plant to be considered an adaptogen, it must meet three criteria:

- Be safe and non-toxic
- Be able to increase our resilience to stress
- Support our health holistically, i.e. not simply by supporting one particular organ, but by helping the whole body/mind achieve a state of balance (termed "homeostasis")

Adaptogens can be thought of as an elite class of plant medicine that supports us in maintaining balance – and thus health – regardless of external circumstances. And, indeed, they go even further by having the capacity to enhance our energy, stamina, endurance and mental clarity, too. Additionally, they are incredibly helpful in improving libido, sexual performance and general enjoyment of life.

It is particularly interesting that most adaptogens that are in common use today hail from thousands of years of use in Traditional Chinese Medicine and Ayurveda – and in both these traditions healthy sexuality was considered to be a cornerstone of robust longevity. Nowadays, there is a whole field of scientific research that backs this up!

How Adaptogens Work

Think of the thermostat in your home that reacts to changes in ambient temperature and acts to bring your home's temperature up or down to the level that you desire. Adaptogens are a little like this. It is intriguing how one herb can, for example, not just lower unhealthily high blood pressure but also raise unhealthily low blood pressure – returning them to normal levels. Similarly, adaptogens can both help you feel more energetic when you are exhausted and calm you down when you are too wired.

Some herbalists view this ability to be a form of plant "intelligence". But, the question remains – why would plants evolve to do this? According to ethnobotanist James Duke, PhD, plants have to contend with lots of stressors themselves, so they developed this adaptogenic ability to survive. It is interesting to note that the most effective adaptogens actually come from some of the harshest environments in the world.

We don't know exactly how adaptogens work, but research shows that they bring balance by acting on the following:

- Stress-hormone production and adrenal function
- Neurotransmitter production and deployment
- Inflammatory response
- Energy levels and blood-sugar metabolism

My Top Five Recommendations

Here follows a countdown of my top five adaptogens to rewind your body clock. Take notice of the Latin names to be sure that you're getting a remedy from the right plant species. Don't rely on common names alone, as they vary widely; for example, there is much confusion among ginsengs.

5. Asian Ginseng (*Panax ginseng*)

Ginseng is one of the most popular herbal remedies with a 5,000-year history of use. Ginseng's botanical name *panax* means "panacea" or "cure-all". Ginseng is used to improve depression, cognitive performance, sleep, energy, sexual function and immunity. Ginseng is the most stimulating of the adaptogens, but because of this it can make anxiety and insomnia worse in some people. If that's the case, you might want to try ginseng's close relative "American ginseng" (see below).

4. American Ginseng (*Panax quinquefolius*)

American ginseng was used as a healing tonic by several Native American tribes including the Cherokee and Iroquois. It has a proven ability to enhance cognitive function. Since it's considered less stimulating than Asian ginseng, it is also a particularly good choice for anxiety relief. I find it really useful if my mind starts to race – as it often can when we just have too many things to do.

3. Siberian Ginseng – AKA Eluthero (*Eleutherococcus senticosus*)

Siberian ginseng has been used as a general health tonic for vigour, stamina and to treat respiratory conditions for over 2,000 years in China. Although it has different active components, its benefits are very similar to those of Asian ginseng, so simply source whichever one is more readily available near you. This herb is also popular in Russia, where it's often used to help people in physically demanding situations. For example, Olympic athletes use it as a natural way to enhance performance and aid training recovery.

2. Ashwagandha (*Withania somnifera*)

One of the key herbs in Ayurvedic medicine, *ashwagandha* literally means "smell of the horse". It is said to "bestow the strength and stamina of a horse" on those who use it. All adaptogens lower stress levels, but ashwagandha excels in this area. It has been found to reduce stress and anxiety by 44 per cent, while decreasing the stress hormone cortisol by 28 per cent. Studies show that it can significantly improve anxiety, depression and insomnia, as well as increase productivity. This is an excellent choice if you're looking for a herb to enhance your overall quality of life.

1. Arctic Root (*Rhodiola rosea*)

Arctic root hails from cold, northern regions of the world and has played an important role in both traditional Scandinavian and Chinese medicine. It was used by the Vikings to increase physical and mental stamina and is currently one of the adaptogens being most widely appreciated for its ability to increase physical vitality. It is unparalleled for overcoming fatigue and exhaustion due to prolonged stressful situations. It can help with depression by transporting serotonin precursors into the brain. It's also a useful aid when you want to quit caffeine since it can minimize withdrawal side effects. I often prescribe Arctic root for patients of mine who are recovering from conditions such as adrenal fatigue, chronic fatigue syndrome, fibromyalgia and burnout.

Note: As with all recommendations in this book, check with a qualified professional (in this case a herbalist) if in any doubt as to a substance's suitability for you. Remember, it's possible to be fine eating a particular food but then find you react to it on your skin, or vice versa. The recommendations have, of course, all been used for many years, but we all react differently to things, so it's always good to err on the side of caution.

REWIND PRACTICE – OVER TO YOU
Try My Healing Salve

Below is my favourite herbal recipe for a healing balm that is fantastic to make your skin both look and feel younger. It is particularly useful if you ever find yourself with rough, chapped skin. This recipe makes 500ml (17oz) of salve, so you'll need a few small jars in which to store it.

400g (14oz) unrefined organic coconut oil
150g (5oz) unrefined food-grade cocoa butter
60g (2oz) fresh herbs of your choice. I use approximately 40g (1.5oz / $^2/_3$ cup) of plantain leaves – these are the little roundish leaves that commonly grow amongst grass, not to be confused with the banana-like plantain (same name but totally different plant) and 20g (0.70oz) of lavender flowers – pick these fresh in summer and hang them to dry so that you have a stash to use all year.
Slow cooker, dehydrator or crock pot – ensure you can set this quite low
Thermometer

1. Put the coconut oil and cocoa butter into the slow cooker or other appliance, and allow to melt completely.
2. Add your plants (plantain and lavender, or see right for a list of other herb options) and ensure that they are totally covered by the oil by squashing them down if necessary. As the oil warms up, they will soften and sink in, but feel free to help them along at the beginning.
3. Using your thermometer to check the temperature, increase the heat so that the plants are cooking at between 37.7 and 60°C (100 and 140°F) for 2–3 hours. Monitor the temperature periodically so that the plants don't get overcooked and go crispy.
4. Your liquid should end up a lovely green colour. Take it off the heat and strain the liquid into your jars.
5. Squeeze your plants once the oil has cooled down so that you get every last drop of healing essence.
6. Allow the jars to cool at room temperature. You might want to help this process by putting the jars in the fridge so the balm hardens up a bit.

7. Once the oil has hardened, bring the jars back out of the fridge for 30 minutes or so to allow the balm to come to the right texture.
8. Store your balm in a cool place so that it doesn't become liquid. However, if this happens, don't worry, just pop it back into the fridge. It should last for about 2–3 months.

Note: It's best to do a patch test of the salve by rubbing a little behind your ear and waiting 24 hours to check for any reactions before using elsewhere.

Other herbs that can be used to make this healing salve include:

- Meadowsweet: An anti-inflammatory herb, its gentle flowers were traditionally used in love potions as it was linked to peace and happiness.
- Calendula: Also an anti-inflammatory and a healing herb par excellence, it works wonders for sunburn, eczema or heat rash.
- Chamomile: Wonderful in a beauty balm, it is also a potent stress reliever.
- Lavender: Fabulous for stress relief and a great sleep aid too.
- Rosemary: Perfect to use when studying, it enhances cognitive performance and memory.
- Sage: An effective herb for inflammatory conditions including arthritis, gout or anything affecting the cardiovascular system. Also a potent cognitive enhancer as it inhibits the enzyme that breaks down one of the brain's chemical messengers, acetylcholine. Use it with rosemary for an extra memory boost, as they each work slightly differently so will support each other's effects.
- Mint: Refreshing and uplifting, this supports memory so could also be used with rosemary and sage.
- Ginger: Excellent for aches and pains, but not on sensitive areas as it can feel hot and prickly.
- Capsicum: Again, not for use on sensitive areas, but ideal together with ginger for use on sore joints.

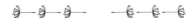

Your Herbs Mindset Moving Forward:
Now that you've come to the end of this chapter, take a little time to think about its content and come up with a specific, positive, present-tense Mindset Phrase of your own for the topic in hand, focusing on the information that has resonated most with you from the chapter.

CHAPTER 11

BREATHE

❝ I use the power of my breath to cultivate vital energy and vibrant health – for my body, mind, emotions and spirit. ❞

One of the most important steps you can take to enhance your health-span, and potentially your lifespan, is learning to breathe properly, as it is your instant access to relaxation, rejuvenation, healing and an enhanced sense of connection. The type of breathing that I'm going to share with you in this chapter is so powerfully holistic that it has even been shown to make skin look more youthful, too.

Breathing is, of course, something we do quite unconsciously, for the most part. When we are born, we have a very natural breath, and if you watch a baby sleeping, you'll see that it breathes from its belly. As we get older and more prone to stressors in our lives, we can often find that we transition toward taking more shallow, "upper-chest" breaths.

The Effects of Stress on Our Breathing

Even though I'm so keenly aware of the importance of correct breathing and I teach breathwork on my retreats – as it is one of the most valuable life skills – I often find that, if I'm under pressure, my shoulders will be up around my ears and my breathing becomes incredibly shallow.

This response is common and is a sign of our body preparing to mount what is called a "fight-or-flight" response – in order to keep it safe from any potentially dangerous stressors, whether real or imagined.

Since training to become a Zen meditation teacher in 2014, I'm even more aware of my breath. So where I might have carried on regardless previously without even realizing the bad habits I was slipping into, I can now more easily detect tell-tale stress signs, such as my shoulders being up and my breathing being shallow, and these act as triggers for me to stop and do some conscious longevity breathing. I hope that this chapter will provide you with a set of techniques that you can return to time and again, when you need a sense of calm, deep connection and relaxation.

Different Breathing Techniques

There are many different types of breathwork associated with different ancient spiritual traditions. The chances are that you'll have come across some of these if you've ever taken yoga or meditation classes. For example, the tradition of *pranayama*, or yogic breathing, is central to the Indian holistic concept of health, and there are many different forms of *pranayama*, which are used for a variety of purposes. However, in this chapter, we will focus on a technique known as Taoist Longevity Breathing, which has its historical roots in Vedic scripture. Just to clarify, Taoism is not a religion – more of a philosophy for a happy, healthy life, with vibrant longevity as one of its central tenets.

The Benefits of Taoist Longevity Breathing

Firstly, let's look at the key benefits of Taoist Longevity Breathing before I move on to teach you some of the specific exercises proven to reduce stress, which in turn will reduce inflammation and our susceptibility to all the largely avoidable chronic diseases associated with ageing.

Taoist Longevity Breathing techniques go far beyond simply improving our ability to take in more oxygen. The focus is on rejuvenating our lungs and other internal organs by reducing the damage associated with AGEs (see Chapter 2), given that these cause the stiffening of proteins (especially collagen), which, in turn, causes not only wrinkles but also potential damage to our eyes, kidneys, lungs, heart, blood vessels and more.

Furthermore, Taoist Longevity Breathing enhances our circulation due to the "pumping action" it requires us to make with our diaphragm. It also boosts our resilience and assists us with processing negative emotions such as fear and anger more effectively due to the way it activates our parasympathetic nervous system (also sometimes called the "rest and digest" part of our nervous system, as it is this part that allows us to relax and conserve energy). This activation creates an internal state that is the opposite to the hyper-adrenalized "fight-or-flight" state mentioned earlier.

Lastly, because the effects of Taoist Longevity Breathing are entirely holistic, it also improves our *overall* fitness, in some cases even contributing to enhanced sports performance. This is possible because we are calmer, less inflamed, better oxygenated and are able to recover more quickly.

Key Insights into Taoist Longevity Breathing

Before giving you the practical guidance, I feel I should mention that Taoist Longevity Breathing can feel a little counterintuitive at first in that your *lungs* don't actively control your air intake while you're doing it. Instead, this technique comprises a set of progressive exercises that activate all parts of your *abdomen*: first lower, then middle, then upper. Doing this allows you to smooth out your breath so that it becomes more even. Eventually you will find that it becomes easier and more natural to slow and extend your breath.

Down the line, if you decide to study with an expert trainer, you'll go on to learn how to activate other areas of your body too, which will increase the effectiveness of the practice. It is said that the study of Taoist Longevity Breathing is a lifelong pursuit as you can go deeper and deeper into the technique, getting progressively more from it.

One of the most important concepts to consider when doing Taoist Longevity Breathing is diaphragmatic control. The diaphragm is a sheet of muscle at the bottom of your ribcage that separates your lungs from your entire abdomen. It wraps around the lower parts of your ribcage and attaches to your spine, and it moves up and down when you breathe.

When you are at rest, or have exhaled, the muscle is bell-shaped. When you breathe in, the muscle flattens and, due to the vacuum that this causes, air is drawn into your lungs. When you breathe out, your diaphragm relaxes and becomes bell-shaped once again, your chest gets smaller, and this causes the air to be pushed out of your lungs.

Diaphragm mobility and strength is very important for overall health, not just from the perspective of breathing, but also for other parts of your anatomy as ligaments link your diaphragm to your internal organs, which causes them to move as you breathe. Ultimately, then, our breath can be thought of as providing a form of internal massage, as if our diaphragm moves well, our internal organs should also be able to move properly – and this will assist with the flow of lymph throughout our body, allowing effective detoxification and therefore encouraging good all-round health. Lymph is a fluid that moves through channels helping to remove accumulated debris from the body. It has no pump as such – unlike our vascular system, through which blood flows due to being pumped around by the heart. Instead, lymph transport relies on our movement and breathing, and the movement of our diaphragm assists with this. (You'll read more about the lymph channels in Chapter 13.)

REWIND PRACTICE – OVER TO YOU
Taoist Longevity Breathing

As just discussed, Taoist Longevity Breathing exercises will help you breathe more healthily, which in turn will improve every function of your body and mind. But it is crucial to learn the techniques slowly and not to force anything, as to do so might stress internal organs.

It can be useful to think of the technique as a dance – focusing on rhythm and transitions between each breath. The power of the practice comes from the smoothness and regularity of the breathing, rather than the amount of breath you can take in or expel, or the amount of time you can hold your breath. In this way, you will be focusing on one of the most important tenets of Taoism: the idea of simply "allowing". Ideally, try to devote at least 10–15 minutes a day to this practice.

1. Inhalation: Begin by flaring your nostrils as you inhale and draw air deep into the base of your lungs. In doing so, observe the way that your abdomen distends. When your lower lungs feel full, continue to inhale very gently and smoothly, allowing your ribcage to expand – and this will fill the middle part of your lungs. Next, inhale a little further to fill your lungs just a little more. Remember not to force your inhalation beyond a comfortable level. About two-thirds full is the right measure. Lastly, visualize "sinking" the breath gently down into your abdominal cavity. This will cause the abdominal wall to balloon out. If you find this difficult, it can help to swallow.

2. Breath Retention: The next step is to hold your breath still for a few seconds after you've inhaled completely and allowed your breath to sink. Begin with a retention of 3–5 seconds – gradually working up, over a period of weeks or months of practice, to a retention of 7–10 seconds. This breath retention will allow your heartbeat to slow down, your blood pressure to be reduced and cellular respiration to be improved.

3. Exhalation: Gently allow your lungs to empty in the reverse order from the inhalation: beginning at the top and ending at the bottom. When

you finally exhale completely, pull your belly in and this will push your diaphragm upward. It helps to think of it as sucking your belly in while you exhale. Again – be sure to do this all very gently.

4. Pause: Once your lungs are empty, close off your glottis at the back of your throat to prevent the air from rushing back into the vacuum left in your lungs. At this point, pause for a few seconds to allow both your abdominal wall and your diaphragm to relax, and then gently start your next inhalation.

You might notice that you get hotter when doing this exercise. In fact, you might even perspire after 10–15 minutes. It is thought that increased cellular respiration is responsible for this. Taoists see it as an increase in *qi*, meaning energy activity.

Once you are used to it, this technique can be incorporated into your daily life in various ways, so experiment to see what suits you best. For example:

• While doing daily activities, like washing the dishes or showering. This can provoke a mindful and calm state and really help you to "be" in the moment.
• As punctuation points of calm throughout the day based on pre-specified triggers, so, for example, when I'm writing I will practise a few rounds of breathing each time I finish a paragraph. Have a think about the kinds of triggers that you can set up that will be meaningful to you.
• As part of your meditation practice: it provokes an excellent mind/body connection and helps you to instantly feel calmer.
• At the end of the day to help you sleep. If I've had a very brain-oriented day – perhaps where I've had to trawl through tons of research papers or analyse statistical research, and my brain won't switch off as fast as I'd like it to, I find a few rounds of Taoist Longevity Breathing works absolute wonders. And if I wake during the night, another few rounds send me right back to sleep!

Your Breathing Mindset Moving Forward:
Now that you've come to the end of this chapter, take a little time to think about its content and come up with a specific, positive, present-tense Mindset Phrase of your own for the topic in hand, focusing on the information that has resonated most with you from the chapter.

CHAPTER 12
VIBRANT EXERCISE

❝ Exercise strengthens me and improves the way that I function in all ways, physically, mentally and emotionally. I get happier, stronger, leaner and more flexible each time I exercise. ❞

There's no doubt about it – exercise, of the right kind, can easily add years of happy, healthy, youthful vibrancy to your life. In fact, exercise is probably one of the most underrated anti-ageing panaceas there is. In this chapter, I'm going to help you work out which exercise strategies are best for you on every level.

Cultivating an Exercise Mindset

As per at the start of every chapter, you have been given a positive mindset nudge via the statement in quotation marks above. However, in my experience, the mindset aspect might be even more important for this chapter than for others so that any exercise you do doesn't become a chore that you do "because you have to" or "because it is in your interest" – but rather something that you do because you are actively developing a loving, nurturing relationship with yourself so that you can be at your very best in all ways. Remember: our body and mind are inextricably interlinked, so our beliefs have an immediate effect on our body – and vice versa.

Thought Experiment

To illustrate how our thoughts alone can have a direct and immediate effect upon our body, just try this simple exercise: Close your eyes and imagine that you are holding a fresh, bright yellow lemon in your hands.

What colour and shape is it? How heavy is it? In your mind's eye, examine the lemon from all sides. Imagine the texture of the skin. Take a knife and cut into it – does a drop of juice spurt out? Cut right through the lemon and squeeze the juice into your mouth. Notice the sharpness and tang. What else do you notice?

By now, I would be really surprised if your mouth wasn't watering! Mine is, and I'm just writing about the exercise. I love this thought experiment because it is such a simple illustration of our physiological response to a thought. While the lemon illustration is quite simplistic, it is helpful as it is a way of understanding that everything we think is noted, measured and reacted to by our bodies. It is therefore super important to be aware of what's going on in our minds (our "self-talk") when we exercise – and also when we think about the way we look and feel.

Do you recall an earlier example of the way that thoughts can directly affect our bodies? On page 60, I mentioned an experiment in which people were asked to visualize exercise rather than actually doing it – and those people got nearly the same gains in strength as people who actually exercised physically. Granted, physical exercise done in isolation can help with all-round wellbeing, so you definitely could just read through this chapter, go and do some sustained exercise over a period of time and get measurably improved fitness results. However, if you add in the mindset dimension too, your results will be all the more incredible!

Arnold Schwarzenegger once said, "Put your mind in your muscle." He knew long before all the fancy neurophysiological research we have today that if you connect thoughtfully to what you are doing, you will reap far better results than just going through the motions. So do bear this in mind as you read on.

The Need for Movement

Our bodies have evolved over millennia in order to facilitate movement: we humans are upright, walking creatures and we developed this way so that we could more easily wander long distances to forage for sustenance. If we don't keep moving, we very quickly succumb to a wide variety of problems, including fat accumulation, changes in body composition (muscle-to-fat ratio), weakness, immune problems and much more. In short, if we don't exercise in one form or another, we age much more quickly and prematurely. One of the easiest ways of staving off the many problems associated with ageing is through exercise – or at least *not* leading a sedentary lifestyle.

Rewind Insight: Fascinatingly, scientists in two separate experiments have discovered that saying swear words while exercising can increase physical performance by between 4 and 8 per cent, depending on the exercise! Research psychologists claim that it is connected to a form of emotional release that appears to allow people to express a specific feeling strongly. However, Richard Stephens, who works at Keele University in England, says that profanities seem to serve a more physical purpose. Stephens and his research colleagues discovered that the improved performance could be explained by the swearing helping with pain management (which makes sense when we think about how people often swear when they hurt themselves). The technique certainly wouldn't be to everyone's tastes! But if you like the idea, a 4–8 per cent gain in something like weightlifting, sprinting or running a long-distance race could be pretty astounding, so feel free to try it!

Combatting the Dangers of Sitting

British researchers have linked prolonged periods of sitting to a greater likelihood of disease – with the caveat that the damage caused by these long periods of sitting were not offset by exercise, including strenuous exercise. So, for example, even if you go and completely "beast yourself" in the gym, but then you go into work and sit down without moving all day, all that work you did in the gym is irrelevant! A team of Australian researchers backed up these findings, reporting that each hour spent watching TV is linked to an 18 per cent increase in the risk of dying from cardiovascular disease – perhaps because that time is spent sitting down!

The health risks of spending too much time just sitting are so apparent now that many companies are investing in "standing desks". And while this trend may not have made it to your workplace or you may not feel it's for you, it really is vital for your health that you at least get up from your desk or work station at regular intervals during the day and move about. Not only will it help to protect you from the diseases associated with sitting, it will also dramatically increase your creativity and productivity, as well as enhancing your mood and generally making you feel better. I suggest setting a timer to go off every 25 minutes to remind you to get up and move for at least a few minutes in every half-hour. Try it and see how you feel! Or start with a few minutes every hour if this feels like too much!

Enhancing Mood

One of the most profoundly anti-ageing effects of exercise is its ability to dramatically lift our spirits. And, as we all know, an improved mood contributes to a greater likelihood that we will be more able, and willing, not only to exercise *more*, but also to do all the other things necessary for a healthier, more vibrant life. And while we *know* this deep down, I think there is an unacknowledged problem in that a lot of people, some health experts included, seem to forget this when giving health advice.

It stands to reason that it's much easier to exercise, eat healthily, get regular sleep etc. when you feel good. There, I said it! It really does often feel like the elephant in the room. When you aren't feeling that great, on the other hand, less constructive behaviours tend to creep in. I personally find that if I get a bit down and feel low – and let's face it, we all do from time to time – my health-promoting behaviours just aren't on point. So, I won't eat as well as I normally do, I might skip supplements, and I probably won't visit friends. Instead, I might well do a Netflix binge, lying on the sofa, eating dark chocolate, stroking my cat. And this is where mindset can make all the difference!

Doing this is fine – and enjoyable – now and again, of course, in order to "switch off". We just need to be careful that it doesn't become an unhealthy pattern. Luckily, I find that I can snap out of a lethargic slump pretty rapidly – probably because I have the advantage of knowing that you have to break the vicious circle and make a change – *any* change – in order to disrupt the pattern.

My "trick" is to force myself to just go out for a brief walk, although you should decide for yourself what would work best for you. It takes a lot of will power, but just this one thing can be done. And once you can muster that simple disruption, you'll find that the wellbeing ball is rolling again and you'll be able to get back on track with everything else, exercise included, more easily. And then, once you're back on track with your exercising, you'll begin to produce all those motivating messenger hormones once again, which will help to keep the momentum going.

A Natural Antidepressant

Regular physical activity has also been correlated with dramatic improvement in clinical depression, anxiety and insomnia. Plus it helps us to become more immune to the effects of stress in the first place as it enhances our overall resilience. And people who become, or remain, physically fit or active have been shown to be less likely to develop clinical depression in the future – even if they have previously suffered from it.

Major studies have shown that vigorous exercise can be as effective as antidepressant medications or cognitive behavioural therapy (CBT), which are standard treatments for depression. However, of course, exercise doesn't have the negative side effects of some medication (such as SSRIs etc.), plus its effects seem to be more immediate.

The antidepressant effect of exercise can be further enhanced if we exercise outside. There are several reasons for this: an external environment provides a changing, thus stimulating, backdrop to our activities, and if we can get out into nature, there are a whole host of beneficial bacteria that we come into contact with that actually alter our body chemistry and make us happier. (See Chapter 17 for more on this.)

Improving Muscle-to-Fat Ratio

Your body composition measurement is important as it gives you an indication of your muscle-to-fat ratio – as well as some insight regarding how your fat is distributed around your body. It is entirely possible to have a high level of body fat but to actually weigh quite little on the scales – and there's even a term for this: "skinny-obese".

I experienced this myself when I was recovering from my illness. My weight had risen to 112lbs (8 stone/51kg) on the scales and I looked very slim, so I thought I was pretty healthy given I was recovering from a devastating illness. However, when I was assessed on a high-tech body composition monitor, to my horror, it showed that my body-fat percentage was dangerously high – basically because I'd been totally immobile for such a long time that my muscle mass had deteriorated dramatically. So, at just 112lbs and a petite UK size 8, I was, technically, obese!

It's really helpful to know your body-fat percentage, as this offers more insight into your overall health than *just* your weight. Carrying too much fat poses a major health risk and ages you rapidly – whether you're overweight or a healthy weight with a high body-fat percentage. Developing an improved muscle-to-fat ratio lowers the risk of all chronic, lifestyle-related and totally preventable diseases.

There are various ways to measure your body-fat percentage, but the most reliable is to get measured by an expert at a sports clinic. I find that domestic scales that claim to be able to measure body composition are very inaccurate and give a variety of measurements throughout the day – depending on whether you've eaten, how hydrated you are and so on. If you find that you're currently above your ideal body-fat percentage (which the expert should tell you based on established guidelines, a selection of which are given in the box opposite), I would first concentrate on building lean muscle – and the best way to do this is to do resistance training, including lifting weights (see also page 142) no matter what your age, so ask a fitness expert for advice on what will best suit your needs.

In fact, while it used to be thought that we can't grow muscle once we get older – or that muscle growth decreases – this has been shown to be untrue; research on people in their nineties turned that erroneous notion on its head. We can gain muscle and strength at any age.

Many experts recommend reducing 500 calories per day from your diet if your muscle-to-fat ratio is poor. However, I disagree with this. Instead I think we need to eat lots of good, healthy whole foods with excellent sources of plant protein to feed our growing muscles, which, in turn, will speed our metabolism in order to burn off the harmful fat, reduce inflammation – and so the virtuous circle will continue.

Reducing Visceral Fat

Fat was often thought of as just an inert substance that was there to provide us with insulation – and, in the case of fat around the hips, bum and thighs in us women, to provide sustenance for a developing foetus. And researchers have, in fact, found that the quantity of fat around this area directly affects a baby's chances of survival, as well as the child's intelligence.

Professor Will Lassek of the University of Pittsburgh, who undertook the groundbreaking study of why women store fat in these regions, found that these fat deposits contain large percentages of docosahexaenoic acid (DHA). DHA is an "essential omega 3 fatty acid" that is needed for the growth and functional development of the brain in infants. Furthermore, DHA is also required for maintaining normal brain function throughout adulthood. DHA actually improves our cognitive ability, and deficiencies of DHA are associated with shortfalls in learning. So it turns out that female hip, bum and thigh fat really *is* there for a very good reason.

However, things take a sinister turn when fat accumulates around our internal organs in the form of visceral fat, as I have previously mentioned. This is not an inert substance at all and produces all manner of highly toxic chemical compounds that dramatically drive inflammation. It's therefore crucial that we put in place a regular movement and exercise regime for ourselves in order not to let visceral fat build up and cause us all kinds of health problems.

Rewind Insight: "Healthy" body-fat percentages are quite different according to gender and increase slightly as we age. There are lots of sources of these figures online, but below are some of the approximate guidelines for healthy percentages that are published widely.

- Women aged 20–40 should aim for 21–33%; men 8–19%
- Women aged 41–60 should aim for 23–35%; men 11–22%
- Women aged over 60 should aim for 24–36%; men 13–25%

Harnessing the Metabolic Benefits of Muscle

Fascinatingly, lean muscle tissue uses calories 24 hours a day, even when you're sleeping. This can account for about 20 per cent of your daily calorie burn, whereas fatty tissue uses calories amounting to only around 5 per cent. This means that someone with a greater amount of lean muscle will have a higher metabolism than someone of the same weight, height, gender and age who has a higher body-fat percentage. All the more reason to get lifting those weights and be vigilant about what you eat.

A Hormonal Perspective

To get a proper perspective of the relationship between hormones and ageing, we need to talk about what is called the Human Growth Hormone (HGH). This is considered to be "the youth hormone", as it is produced in higher levels when we are growing and drops precipitously at around age 20 – see also the graph overleaf.

Then, when you reach your thirties and beyond, your levels of HGH continue to peter out, which triggers a phenomenon called "somatopause", which is part of what drives your ageing process. It is at this stage that many people start putting on body fat – especially abdominal fat – and losing muscle; we become more tired and lethargic, and the dreaded "middle-age spread" sets in, which makes it all the more important than ever to keep (or start) exercising as we get older.

High levels of HGH are associated with better health overall and researchers say that it supports better body composition because it facilitates greater muscle-to-fat ratio and it is also associated with emotional factors such as feeling more positive and motivated.

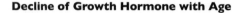

Decline of Growth Hormone with Age

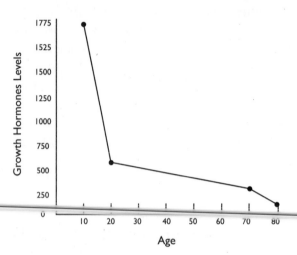

Interestingly, all forms of exercise and movement in themselves contribute to the optimization of the production of HGH. And the longer you can keep your body producing higher levels of HGH, the longer you will experience robust health and strength – both physically and mentally. So finding a form of exercise that you love and are happy to do regularly really is vital to boosting your health-span.

Doing everything else right to rewind your body clock – from eating the right foods, working on your stress-response management, meditating etc. – *without* exercise could be compared to "one-hand clapping". That is to say, not a waste of time, just not entirely fruitful! All researchers agree that, by exercising, you can limit bone and muscle loss as you age. However, there are so many types of exercise to choose from that it can feel difficult to know what the best kind is for you. So let's look now at the key benefits of a range of some of the most popular and beneficial anti-ageing forms of exercise to help you get started.

Choosing the Best Type of Exercise for You

The following are all types of exercise proven to increase production of the Human Growth Hormone just discussed and therefore to help rewind our biological clock. Obviously this is by no means a *comprehensive* list of the types of exercise that you might want to try, but hopefully you will find it a useful starting point for your Rewind explorations.

Vigorous exercise: HIIT
Increasingly, research is looking at the amazing biological age-reversal effects of High Intensity Interval Training (HIIT), whereby you intersperse intense exercise with moderate exercise within one short training session. HIIT is an excellent way of increasing HGH – but only if you avoid carbohydrates for two hours after the session (as soon as you take carbs into your body, the HGH "tap" is turned off).

Research published in the journal *Preventative Medicine* reported that in a study of 5,825 adults in the USA between 1999 and 2002 (known as the "National Health and Nutrition Examination Survey"), those who exercised regularly were markedly younger on a cellular level than those who led sedentary or even reasonably active lifestyles. Participants were asked demographic and lifestyle questions, including how often they exercised, and the researchers also analysed the participants' telomere length against their levels of physical activity. Professor Tucker discovered that people with a high level of physical activity were, biologically, nine years younger than sedentary people.

The intensity of exercise is relevant too. When Professor Tucker compared vigorous exercisers with those who did a moderate amount of exercise, the difference for the highly active people was seven years; in this study, a high level of physical activity was deemed to be running between 30–40 minutes per day, at least five days per week.

We don't know exactly why exercise seems to preserve telomere length, but the current scientific thinking is that it could be linked to a reduction of inflammation and oxidative stress, as exercise suppresses both of these over time.

Moderate Exercise
HIIT is hard – and pretty advanced – but fear not. If you don't fancy doing HIIT sessions, a very recent meta-analysis (overview) of studies in exercise shows that just 30 minutes of moderate exercise can help to prevent 24 chronic diseases. So, happily, vigorous exercise isn't the only way to reverse your biological age. For example, I encourage my patients to walk at a moderate pace for at least 20–30 minutes four times per week, or more often if they can. This is an outstanding strategy for burning off excess body fat (particularly visceral fat) and dramatically improving muscle-to-fat ratio. I have seen "beer bellies" on both men and women (usually related to poor diet, stress, lack of sleep and little exercise, rather than beer by the way!), disappear within weeks.

Resistance Training

Lifting weights – or using your own body weight to exercise (called calisthenics) – is another vital part of our anti-ageing arsenal. So, firstly, let's bust some myths about this. Conventional wisdom has it that women should lift low weights and perform higher repetitions (reps) in order to grow "long, lean muscles". This concept appeals to many women as they don't want to appear bulky or masculine-looking.

However, the truth of the matter is that, on the whole, women simply don't have the hormonal make-up (high enough levels of testosterone) to create bulky muscles. Sure, lifting weights will make your muscles grow – especially if you are lifting heavier weights at fewer reps – but what actually happens is that your body becomes more toned, so:

- You will probably therefore get smaller – especially around the waist and midriff area;
- Your bum will lift;
- Your thighs and arms will tone (begone bingo-wings!);
- And unless you start to do some serious competitive body-building and strip your body fat right down – so that every muscle can be seen clearly – you will simply look (and be) younger, hotter and fitter!

So, what more reason do you need to get down to your local gym and recruit a trainer who knows what they are doing and start to pump some iron? Both your lifespan and health-span will really thank you for it.

Another myth, already briefly mentioned on page 138, is that as we age, we simply can't grow muscle. The truth is that exercise at any age produces astounding results. In the 90+ Study, initiated in 2003 and published in the science journal *Age* (now *Geroscience*) of the American Aging Association, a group of people over the age of 90 were asked to exercise for 12 weeks. This was shown to improve both their muscle mass and power,

Rewind Insight: It's ideal to do some exercise first thing in the morning if you can find, or make, the time, as it spikes brain activity and immunizes you against mental stresses for the rest of the day. It has also been proven to help you retain new information and improve your reaction to complex situations.

as well as leading to an increase in walking speed, improved ability to get out of their chairs, and better balance, which led to a significant reduction in the incidence of falls. The upshot? It's never too late to begin exercising!

Tai Chi

Originally a Chinese martial art, tai chi has been recognized for hundreds of years for its health-promoting advantages, and its anti-ageing benefits in particular. Over the years, hundreds, if not thousands, of studies have shown that this low-impact form of exercise – the aim of which is to enhance the flow of energy (known as *chi*) around the body – can help improve quality of life and support the management of symptoms for those suffering from conditions ranging from insomnia, arthritis, osteoporosis and high blood pressure to breast cancer, cardiovascular disease, Parkinson's, Alzheimer's and much more. Tai chi addresses all the multifaceted constituents of fitness:

- Muscle strength
- Flexibility
- Balance
- Aerobic conditioning

In fact, a study published in the international journal *Cell Transplantation* solidly demonstrates tai chi's remarkable anti-ageing benefits due to the way it boosts our stem cells. Researchers at the Center for Neuropsychiatry at China Medical University Hospital in Taiwan divided 36 participants, all of whom were under the age of 25, into three groups. The first group regularly practiced tai chi for a year, the next group exercised with speed walking for a year, and the third group did no exercise at all.

The researchers were particularly interested in whether tai chi had any effect on stem cells known as CD34+. These cells are involved in many of our body's functions and structures as well as being markers for blood stem cells that help facilitate cell renewal, differentiation (the way that "blank stem cells" turn into other types of cells, e.g. heart, bone, skin, brain etc.), and proliferation (the way that cells multiply and travel to where they are required). Cell renewal is involved in maintaining and repairing many functions of our organ systems, which normally slows with age. In short, then, these CD34+ stem cells are mighty anti-ageing warriors.

Results from the study showed that the group of people who practised tai chi had a dramatically higher number of CD34+ cells than the people who performed no exercise at all: astonishingly, the practice of tai chi raised stem cell counts in increments of three to five times. The scientists who conducted the study also reported that the tai chi boosted participants' heart function, stimulated neural cells in their brains, helped regulate excitement and inhibition controls, and eased the stress of mental trauma and nerve exhaustion. It is interesting to note, however, that there was no major difference between the CD34+ stem cell count in the people who practised tai chi and those who did the speed walking. So, if you don't feel tai chi is your thing, you can always get outside for some brisk walks instead – and gain the benefits of being out in nature, too. If you do like the idea of trying tai chi, though, then just look up local teachers in your area and/or find a reputable teaching source online.

Yoga

Another form of exercise that has been proven to enhance health and vitality in all sorts of ways is the ancient Indian art of yoga, which is now widely practised in many forms in the West.

Daily yoga practice has been shown in studies to increase two key substances that are linked to youth and longevity: Human Growth Hormone (see page 139) and dehydroepiandrosterone sulphate (DHEA-S).

We have already explored how HGH has the power to help rewind your body clock, but we haven't yet discussed DHEA-S – a hormone that is produced in our adrenal glands and is linked to improved immune function and heart health, among other factors.

Many studies have shown that regular exercise brings about increased levels of HGH and DHEA-S throughout our lifespan, and a group of scientists in India decided to test whether this would also relate to regular yoga practice in particular. At the end of the 12-week study, the participants showed significant increases in their blood serum HGH and DHEA-S values, plus their body mass index (or BMI; a key index for relating weight to height) had decreased to more healthy levels.

While this study is by no means a definitive marker for yoga being the fountain of youth, it does suggest that regular intensive yoga practice – for a period of an hour or more – relates to having higher levels of indicators known to be related to cell generation and enhanced health. And even if you can't find the time to dedicate an hour to a yoga practice each day, you'll still reap many of the outstanding benefits of this ancient exercise system if you make a point of doing it regularly and consistently.

The beauty of yoga these days is that there is an abundance of great classes out there, both in person and online, so it's just a matter of finding a style and teacher that you like, whether in the gym, in a yoga studio or in the comfort of your own home – although it's best to have lessons to begin with so that you can be sure your postures are correct, both to prevent injury and enhance your practice.

Sex as an Anti-Ageing Strategy

Another form of exercise worth remembering – and often overlooked in terms of its health-enhancing qualities – is an active sex life. Yes, your healthy life expectancy may be increased through having more sex!

The link between sex and ageing is being taken increasingly seriously by the medical community. In fact, one study focusing on men demonstrated that guys who experience a high frequency of orgasms showed a 50 per cent reduction in mortality. While, for women, sex has been shown to increase production of HGH, which, as we have just seen on pages 139–40, is akin to a dose of the elixir of youth.

As it happens, by the way, men are often studied in this area of research as they don't have the hormonal fluctuations that menstruating women experience throughout the monthly cycle, thus providing clearer results on a more level playing field. But many of the findings apply to women too, of course.

Why sex should be linked to life expectancy is something of a mystery. Of course, it could be that generally healthier people are more likely to have more sex and that the findings linking sex to life expectancy are reflecting this, but I think there is more to it than that.

It is well known in anti-ageing research circles that having good relationships and being positive in outlook are linked to longer life expectancies. Consultant neuropsychologist at the Royal Edinburgh Hospital, Dr David Weeks, who made a ten-year study of the subject, found that improving the quality of one's sex life can help a person to look between four and seven years younger. He explains: "A good sex life leads to greater contentment, significant reductions in stress, better sleep and, in men, an increase in testosterone output."

For his landmark study, Dr Weeks questioned more than 3,500 volunteers throughout the decade of his research into the secrets of youthful appearance and behaviour. He concluded that genetic factors were only 25 per cent responsible for youthful looks, while behaviour was 75 per cent the cause. And one of the main behavioural factors was sex as part of a long-term relationship.

The Rejuvenating Power of the Orgasm

What's more, you don't even have to be in a long-term relationship to reap the anti-ageing benefits of orgasms. Research has shown that no matter how an orgasm comes about, it is still a profoundly youth-promoting phenomenon. Masturbation, therefore, is also a wonderful anti-ageing strategy that has been proven to work!

Orgasms increase the production of a wide range of neurotransmitters that are intrinsically linked to greater confidence, happiness and feelings of wellbeing. Having an orgasm at the start of a migraine can prevent the migraine from developing further, and they can even help to ease menstrual cramps. And orgasms before sleep also have the advantage of promoting better sleep quality and a whole host of youth-promoting benefits derived from optimal sleep (see Chapter 18 for more on this).

Plus, on top of all this, preliminary research hypothesizes that frequent sexual intercourse and orgasms may stimulate brain-cell regeneration and contribute to enhanced performance on memory tests. Several studies appear to indicate that intercourse may contribute to an improved rate of brain-cell survival and/or stimulate new neural development (called neurogenesis) in the hippocampus, the area of the brain that is responsible for learning and memory.

There are a number of theories about why sexual intercourse may have this positive impact on cognitive function, including:

- It is a form of exercise, which is known to be beneficial for brain health
- It decreases stress and depression
- It stimulates "reward" centres in your brain, which reinforces and strengthens memory
- It stimulates the production of serotonin and oxytocin, two neurotransmitters that may promote new neural development and that are also intrinsically linked to enhancing relationships and generally feeling wonderful!

Whatever the reason, more sex seems to provide anti-ageing benefits in every respect – so go for it, and enjoy!

Exercise Specifically for Brain Health

We all know that the well-worn phrase "Use it or lose it!" applies to muscles, but did you know that it also applies to your brain? Of course, brain-training exercises, such as Sudoku and crosswords etc., increase our grey matter, but it turns out that you can actually get an additional brain boost by putting your trainers on and hitting the gym – or even donning your best sequined frock and tripping the light fantastic.

Physical activity – especially aerobic exercise and lifting weights – has been proven to have positive effects on our brain function both on a molecular and behavioural level. In fact, recent research shows that even exercising for 20 minutes can improve our information-processing abilities and support memory function. It is believed that exercise affects our brain in the following ways:

- Increases the heart rate, which pumps more oxygen and nutrients to the brain – giving your brain the fuel it needs to function optimally
- Facilitates the release of a cascade of hormones, all of which support a nourishing environment for the growth of brain cells (neurogenesis), and many of which are feel-good hormones (oxytocin, serotonin etc.), resulting in decreased stress-hormone production
- Increases growth factors in the brain, which actually make it easier for the brain to grow new connections (neuroplasticity)
- Boosts cell growth in the hippocampus – the area of the brain that is responsible for learning and memory (the hippocampus is sometimes called "the brain's brain")

There are lots of brain-training apps and online resources that are inexpensive and easy to access. They are definitely worth trying as part of the quest to rewind your body clock as they really do help to improve cognitive function, which will ultimately result in our brains working better for longer and hopefully staving off dementia.

However, if you want to really ensure your brain health into old age, physical exercise is also absolutely essential. It used to be thought that our cognitive function declines automatically as we get older, but nothing could be further from the truth. Older brains do behave a little differently – for example, as we age it may take us slightly longer to learn "new tricks". However, our ability to learn is not compromised overall, which means we can make dramatic improvements to our cognitive function very quickly.

In fact, using physical exercise *alongside* brain-stimulation methods increases our chances of improving cognitive function even further. Our brains have been proven to thrive on novelty – so, for example, we will get more brain health benefit from getting out and cycling in a changing landscape than from running repetitively on a treadmill, as the brain will have more stimulation to continuously engage with on a mental level.

The Most Effective Form of Brain Exercise

Most researchers agree that the best brain anti-ageing activity that you can do is dancing – and in particular ballroom dancing. This is because it is an activity that has both physical and mental demands, as well as providing valuable social interaction, which has been shown to add approximately nine healthy years to your lifespan (see Chapter 16 for more on this).

Ballroom dancing involves the integration of lots of different parts of our brains in order to master a combination of coordination, response to rhythm, both following and *remembering* choreography, working with a partner and spatial awareness when on the dancefloor – all of which add up to having a superior impact on our cognitive functioning over just physical or mental exercise alone.

In Summary

Ultimately, whatever your age, it is vital to incorporate a variety of different exercise styles into your life. So whether you like to dance, walk, run, lift weights, do tai chi, practise yoga, have sex, do HIIT workouts (if you are fit enough) or whatever else, just do it! And don't just do one. Instead, choose a balance of several different forms. And be mindful that you can lose a lot of the benefits of exercising if you then spend too much time sitting at your desk or in front of the TV or computer. So keep moving! And enjoy!

Your Exercise Mindset Moving Forward:

Now that you've come to the end of this chapter, take a little time to think about its content and come up with a specific, positive, present-tense Mindset Phrase of your own for the topic in hand, focusing on the information that has resonated most with you from the chapter.

REWIND PRACTICE – OVER TO YOU
Let's Get Moving!

Here follows a little guidance to help you find a balance of exercise types that gives you all the qualities you need for a long, healthy life in the form of strength, flexibility, balance, aerobic capacity (the ability of the heart and lungs to get oxygen to the muscles) and enhanced brain health, too.

I encourage you to explore as many different kinds of exercise as possible until you find a combination that you really enjoy, so that you're more likely to stick at it! After all, it's longevity that we're looking for here!

It's important to remember that rest is as crucial for optimal fitness as exercise. Otherwise, you risk overtraining, injury and exhaustion. So please note that the timing suggestions below are only a starting point for you (see also pages 227–8 of the 21-Day Rewind Plan for more guidance on potential ways to structure your exercise throughout the week). There's no need to exercise every day. In fact, it's good to take "rest" days, so be sure to listen and respond to what your body tells you.

- Aim to do resistance training three (or up to four) times a week, ensuring you don't train the same muscle sets on consecutive days. This might include lifting weights, so it's best to initially get help from a trainer if you're new to it, as correct form is essential to avoid injury and to tone up most efficiently.
- Explore forms of exercise that work on flow and flexibility, such as tai chi, yoga, Pilates and qi gong. These are also great for enhancing your body–mind connection. Ideally do one of these activities at least three times a week (if not more).
- Look for activities that raise your heart rate (check online for optimal heart rates for different age groups) and that have the potential to get you out of breath – just enough so that you can still hold a conversation but you'll probably be sweating. Aim to do this about three times a week.
- Explore activities that include an element of variety, such as circuit training due to the mix of exercises, or an element of multi-tasking, such as dancing, as these work *lots* of areas in the brain as well as the body.
- Always gauge the level of exercise that is appropriate for you in terms of not only duration and regularity, but also intensity – and seek advice from a fitness professional if you are unsure.

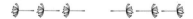

CHAPTER 13

LOOKING YOUNGER NATURALLY

« I care for myself with love and kindness, and nurture my appearance, making the best choices that support my growth toward natural youthfulness, energy and vibrancy. »

In this chapter we're going to get really practical with ways you can help yourself look younger, healthier and more vibrant – on the *outside*. I've shared these over the years with my patients to fabulous effect – and I can't wait to share them with you!

There will be no need to go under the knife once you have these techniques down. Firstly, you'll find suggestions about both nutrition and hydration for optimal skin. Next, we'll look at some natural lotions and remedies to use on the skin. Then you'll find a range of top beauty hacks to help you stay looking young. And finally you'll be given step-by-step guidance for three complete facial exercise routines: a four-step natural face-lift routine; a specially designed lymphatic drainage facial; and a Chinese acupressure facial routine. Note that the latter three approaches aren't meant to be done directly after one another, so just follow the notes on page 169 for when it's best to do each one.

Our Skin as a Barometer of Health

The condition of our skin is an excellent barometer for how we are doing internally, so while having great skin may, at first, seem to be only a cosmetic concern, taking good care of it is actually a very useful health strategy.

Women tend to have a harder time of it skin-wise than men because female skin is thinner and thus more prone to wrinkling and, of course, hormonal fluctuations, which can cause all sorts of problems ranging from acne to premature wrinkling. The good news, though, is that there is a lot we can do to enhance our skin and keep it looking as vibrant as possible.

Eating Well

On a personal note, I have noticed that since I switched to a plant-based, wholefood diet about 11 years ago, my skin has dramatically improved. To my amazement, I have actually seen wrinkles disappear, especially on my forehead, where they were quite deep before. In addition to the general nutritional guidance in Chapter 6, when it comes to my quest for glowing skin, I try to eat as much raw, living food as possible. Sprouted seeds and legumes are great, so I often add sprouted sunflower, broccoli, alfalfa and more to my meals. Whether your entire diet is plant-based or not, try sprinkling them on salads, for example.

These foods punch way above their weight nutritionally, with outstanding health and beauty benefits. We're only just beginning to understand, scientifically, why they are so good for us and why they seem to have such a big influence on our looks, and skin health in particular: as well as being full of high-quality protein, they are at an incredibly energetic part of the plant's growth cycle and appear to have incredible levels of enzymes that are beneficial to us humans. More answers will no doubt emerge from the field of nutrigenomics, which involves scientists attempting to understand how foods affect the expression of certain genes.

Ditching Sugar

Avoiding refined sugar is one of the best ways of reducing any bloating around the face – and elsewhere in the body. If you've heard the term "carb face", you'll already know that refined carbohydrates are the main culprits of this phenomenon because they cause water retention. Biscuits, cakes, breads and pasta are all generally high in processed grains and sugars, and for every gram of carbohydrate, your body will retain 3–5g of water. In addition, it's best to steer clear of snack foods like crisps (chips), which are full of salt and also contribute to water retention.

This all adds to the argument for following a plant-based, wholefood diet, as this way of eating is undeniably low in simple carbohydrates. Plus, when we eat this way, we're not subjecting ourselves to the ravages of AGE exposure, which, as we know from page 42, wreaks havoc both internally and externally, ageing us dramatically. However, even if you're not ready to go fully plant-based with your diet, you can make a big difference to the quality of your skin by starting to cut down on all forms of refined carbohydrate in your diet.

Staying Hydrated: The Importance of Water

Adequate hydration is vital to younger, more vibrant-looking skin. Ensuring that you drink sufficient quantities of water throughout the day will help with the elimination of toxins from your body, thus making your skin look brighter for sure. Water has the added advantage of helping our brains work efficiently, too.

REWIND PRACTICE – OVER TO YOU
Hydrating for Youthful Skin

Below are some suggestions to help you stay hydrated on a daily basis. It's especially important to do these things on busy days as these are the times when it's easiest to neglect our own most fundamental needs.

- Drink a glass of warm water with lemon every morning to kickstart your day (see also page 73)
- Carry a bottle of filtered water with you at all times during the day, and/or keep a jug of water nearby so that you can gradually sip away at it, preventing yourself from becoming dehydrated.
- It's best not to drink during meals as it can cause digestive difficulties; instead take fluid on board half an hour or so before or after meals.
- Check the colour of your pee now and again when you go to the toilet: ideally, it should be a very light straw colour.
- If ever you find yourself raiding the cupboards for a snack, try having a glass of water first; sometimes, we mistakenly think we're hungry when we're actually thirsty!
- Check in with yourself about 15 minutes before bed to see if you're thirsty. If so, have a cup of calming herbal tea, such as chamomile. Don't drink too much before bed, though, in case it makes you need to get up to pee!

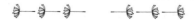

The Value of Cleansing

Cleansing, before moisturizing, is one of the most fundamentally important things you can do for your skin. Once in a while, shop-bought face wipes are fine, especially if you're travelling, for example. However, for daily use, ideally both morning and night, it's best to try to find a simple, organic cleansing lotion that you apply and then rinse off with warm (not hot) water. (Hot water strips your skin of its natural oils and can cause dry patches, breakouts and more, as your skin's biological integrity is compromised.) A quality cleansing lotion not only removes all make-up but is a kind approach that won't dry out your skin.

The Power of Moisturizing

Most of us know already that skin moisturization is a must in order to look better on a quick-fix level. But using a good-quality, natural moisturizer both on your face and the rest of your body, daily, has long-term benefits too, as it helps to keep the skin (our largest organ) hydrated and youthful.

It's important to know what you're looking for when choosing anything that will be applied to the skin (called topical treatments in health circles) – and also to be sure that any products you choose don't contain dangerous chemicals such as parabens (see Chapter 15 for more on this). Everyone's skin is different, and even our own sensitivities change from time to time. My rule of thumb is to always read labels and choose products that have the fewest ingredients possible. And if in doubt in terms of product suitability, do a patch test behind your ear, leaving for 24 hours to check for any adverse reactions.

Unleashing Your Inner Glow

I'd now like to share with you a little insight into three skin treatments that I have seen (and that research proves!) work wonders for many people. I like to call these "skin superstars". Remember: always follow the instructions on product labels and do a small patch test behind the ear as explained above before applying any remedies more generously elsewhere.

Retinol

This form of Vitamin A has been around for a while now and is often given on prescription for the treatment of acne. It is being increasingly used to combat wrinkles, too. However, in order for it to really work, you need to get a strength of at least 0.4 per cent. This is usually only available from a dermatologist – or your doctor if you're lucky enough to have a particularly understanding one.

I use a retinol serum from time to time that I bought in the USA. I have to say that I have been extremely impressed with its cosmetic effects. I have noticed that fine lines around my eyes have gone, and deeper lines have improved. The downside? Well, you have to build up your tolerance to Retinol, as it can be harsh on the skin and lead to redness.

Rosehip Oil

This superb product has been shown in trials to really improve the appearance of skin and also to heal scars – as the oils derived from the rose (called *Rosa mosqueta*) contain a special form of vitamin A. Studies on post-surgical scars and other skin defects at the University Hospital of Seville using this oil state that the results "must be considered excellent".

Rosehip oil can be bought at most health food stores and should be used directly on your skin following the instructions on the packaging, as each preparation differs. I use a *Rosa mosqueta* serum twice a day, morning and evening, and have had great results.

Hyaluronic Acid

Hyaluronic acid (HA) is a naturally occurring carbohydrate that is found virtually everywhere in the human body. It has numerous functions, some of which are to bind water, lubricate the movable parts of the body, such as muscles and joints, and maintain the elasticity of the skin. Because HA is one of the most hydrophilic molecules in nature (meaning it has a strong tendency to attract and hold water molecules), it is sometimes referred to as "nature's moisturizer" – and it really can make a difference to skin, plumping out fine lines and wrinkles. Unfortunately, our production of HA decreases as we get older. It can therefore be useful to give ourselves a boost of HA to counteract the effects of ageing.

One way of doing this is to use one of the many commercially available creams, gels or serums containing HA. According to published research, admittedly by cosmetic companies, these HA preparations stimulate the production of collagen and therefore plump up any sagging areas, as well as hydrating the skin by attracting water molecules to the surface.

Alternatively, you can take HA capsules, which are commonly available from many supplement suppliers. This improves skin too, but because you're ingesting the substance, it also appears to have beneficial effects on joints and eye health.

I have actually had HA injections into my knees – to help cushion the joints in an attempt to mitigate some of the damage that years of rheumatoid arthritis has done to my bones and cartilage. These injections definitely did a good job at reducing pain and improving mobility – more so than non-steroidal anti-inflammatories (NSAIDs) such as ibuprofen, for example. The benefits were temporary, as to be expected with rheumatoid arthritis, but I would still recommend them as temporary relief for anyone suffering from debilitating RA symptoms, as they *do* help; and from what I hear, the injections seem to work even better and longer for people with osteoarthritis. If you are suffering from this kind of issue then do check with your doctor to see if you can get a referral for this treatment.

Rewind Insight: Many of the injectable wrinkle "fillers" on the market today use hyaluronic acid (HA; see page 155–6 for more on this substance). The evidence shows that these work well to plump up skin and fill out lines – and they also seem to help increase the production of collagen, in situ. While I wouldn't exactly describe them as entirely "natural", given that, as explained on page 155, the substance used is already present in our bodies, it is not entirely alien either. One of the advantages of having HA fillers is that you walk away from a treatment with an instantly visible result. While I prefer to recommend completely natural approaches, there's a lot to be said for quick, tangible results as they can have a huge impact on self-esteem. Many of my patients report that they have felt so much better after fillers that it has given them the impetus to dedicate more time to looking after themselves in other ways, such as getting to the gym or improving their nutrition.

The art, I think, with fillers is not to go overboard so that you look "done". If you're considering getting these injections, be sure to find an experienced expert and talk to them about the kinds of results they think look great. If you come across someone of the "more is more" way of thinking, I suggest you beat a hasty retreat. Word of mouth is often best, so see what your friends and acquaintances are getting done – and I can pretty much guarantee you that they are, so ask around!

Quick and Easy Beauty Hacks

Next, I'd like to share with you some of my favourite, tried-and-tested, youth-defying beauty hacks, from gorgeous eyes, brows and lashes to luscious lips and teeth to die for.

Eye-Opening Trick

Droopy eyelids and "hooded" eyes can affect us all as we get older, so I'd like to share with you a fantastic eye shadow technique that I was taught by my friend Ariane Poole, celebrity make-up artist to the stars. I call it "doing the 7s" (you'll see why as you read it) and it really works wonders in terms of giving the effect of lifted, more "open" eyes. If you keep your eyes open when you apply the eye shadow, you'll be able to go higher in the eye crease with your contouring colour (the dark colour mentioned in the steps that follow). Just in case you didn't know, a contouring colour is usually a darker colour that doesn't have shiny or light-reflective particles. Using it in the way explained below will help to create depth to the eye, which will help to create the desired illusion of lift.

1. Keeping both eyes open as just mentioned, take a dark colour, such as a dark shade of brown, from the inner part of your eyelid, just below your brow bone, and sweep out toward your brow end.
2. Next use the same colour to sweep upward from the outer upper lid, to meet the end of the first stroke.
3. So, your darker shade should now look like a "7" shape – with the corner of the 7 toward the outer side of your eyelid. (Don't do it the other way around, for goodness sake, as that would look very weird!)
4. Now blend, blend and blend like crazy – for an instant youthful effect!

Beautiful Brows

People tend to have different shape and size preferences when it comes to their eyebrows. However, shaping your brows correctly can knock years off your face, so if you aren't sure which shape will best lift your face, consider getting a one-to-one lesson with a proper brow artist.

In the meantime, however, here are a few top tips to help you manage them better yourself:

• Lay your tweezers against your cheek so that one end is at the bottom of your nose and the other reaches the inner corner of your eye. The point where the tweezers intersect your brow is where you should *start* your eyebrow shaping.

- Then move your tweezers so that the bottom end stays at the bottom of your nose and the other is now at the *outer* corner of your eye. This time the point where the tweezers intersect your brow is where your eyebrow should *end*, so only pluck hairs *beyond* this.
- Ensure that the arch of your brow peaks above the outer rim of your iris, right on your brow bone; generally pluck from the *lower* side of your brows; not from above.
- Make the tail of your brow (beyond the arch) a bit thinner than the main part, tapering at the end.

Lovely Lashes

A good way of taking care of your lashes so they don't get brittle and fall out as you age is dabbing a tiny bit of night cream onto the tips with your fingers before you go to bed, so that they're moisturized while you sleep. Just be careful that you don't get any cream in your eyes as you do this.

Otherwise, you might like to go for what is called a "lash lift" – a treatment that you can get quite easily now in many beauty salons, although it goes under a variety of different trade names in different places. The lash lift is actually a variety of a lash perm, but thankfully it differs dramatically from the old-fashioned type which simply curled your lashes back toward your eyelid, making them actually look *shorter*. Don't worry though, this new "lash lift" technique lifts your lashes up by bending them at the *roots*, so that it really opens the eyes up – with the result of immediately younger-looking, wider awake eyes.

The lady I go to also dyes my eyelashes, which means I can go weeks without needing mascara – a bonus that I would definitely recommend if mascara makes you feel as good as it does me.

Lip Tricks

Full disclosure: I was taught the below invaluable optical trick back in the mid-'80s by the world-famous drag queen, Miss Ruby Venezuela, who, in my humble opinion, was one of the greatest make-up experts to walk the earth. Here's what the divine Miss Ruby told me:

- For those of us with smaller, or more mature lips, avoid dark hues – especially anything matt. Instead, go for softer tones and apply a lighter shade to the middle of the lower lip and also two smaller dots in the same lighter shade near the top of your upper lip, under your cupid's bow, and blend thoroughly. This will give the illusion of plumpness and ultra-kissable lushness.

- Next, use a highlighter – in a light shade that you'd use on your cheekbones to contour your face, for example – just *above* the V of your cupid's bow and blend, blend, blend to give the illusion of lifting your upper lip; this "lift" is synonymous with more youthful-looking lips.

Natural Tooth Whiteners

To look as vibrantly youthful as possible, try never to over-whiten your teeth. It's unlikely that you'd be able to do this with natural approaches anyway, but if you're tempted to get a dentist to whiten your teeth, be cautious. Over-white teeth are often synonymous with the "denture" look – which can, ironically, be tremendously ageing.

Foods containing malic acid – such as strawberries, apples and grapes – make good teeth-whitening snacks, as this gentle acid acts as a natural tooth cleanser, safely breaking down any stains. (Once you've eaten any of these foods, though, it's best to wait an hour before brushing your teeth as acid in foods and drinks can soften your tooth enamel.)

And if you want to make your teeth look even more sparkly, choose lipsticks that are on the more *orange* end of the red spectrum, as this gives the optical illusion of whiter teeth, and, as we know, whiter teeth are often perceived as belonging to younger, healthier people.

More Beauty Top Tips

- To reduce face wrinkles: Sleep wrinkles are the lines that form when your face is compressed against a pillow night after night. They develop in predictable locations based on fixed anchor points that attach your skin to bone. Sleeping on your back prevents their formation and will also give you better back alignment.

- To banish eye bags: Cut down on salt, increase water intake and investigate whether certain foods – such as wheat, dairy or alcohol – may be causing inflammation in the eye area. I know that if I eat wheat, I get incredibly puffy around the eyes.

- To brighten your face: Learn how to use highlighter properly, as a sexy sheen can make skin look healthily taut. Wayne Goss is one person I really admire and trust among many who does amazing YouTube tutorials for us "grown-up" women.

- To help make-up stay on: Always start your routine with a good primer. I get quite oily but a good primer helps my make-up stay put as well as evening out texture. This is really handy if I have to do photo shoots or if I just don't want to look greasy (never attractive!) in meetings.

- To even out skin tone: It's important to get the colour of any foundation or tinted moisturizer right. If you have sun spots, look for a shade between the darker sun spots and the rest of your skin. And, even if you're sun-spot free, use warmer tones, as these will make you look younger. Lastly, don't use powder as it will amplify any lines on your face, unless you're extremely oily, in which case just dab a little on your T-zone, avoiding any wrinkles, so the powder doesn't settle in them.

Facial Exercises

One of the pioneers of facial exercises was the amazing facial fitness expert Eva Fraser, who developed a now-established set of exercises to lift and tone the face. Her theory is that if we can improve the look of our bodies by exercising, then why not our face, too? And she is right. Eva concentrates on strengthening and tightening the muscle groups in the face and neck that slacken as we age, and her work gets astounding results.

I saw Eva only recently and, despite being 90 years of age now, she looks fantastic, with tight, healthy skin. She said to me, "Jayney, you're only 55 – that's still really young. Women like you have a lot to do in this world and you might as well look good doing it, so exercise those muscles – every day!" So, I do! This inspiring lady and her colleagues are shining evidence to me that facial exercises are worth doing – every day.

My Natural Face-Lift Routine

In the pages that follow I present you with a unique set of natural face-lift exercises that I have put together, drawn from many different sources, expanding on Eva's amazing work and inspired by my many years of experience working with private clients. My criteria when choosing the exercises was that they all needed to be easy to learn, quick to do (in order to fit into your busy life), safe and, of course, effective!

The exercises I'm going to teach you are quite demanding – but that's a good thing! Of all the exercises out there, you'll get the quickest results from these. This is because they are "compound exercises" that also incorporate "resistance training". So, rather like doing squats, or planking, they don't just isolate and target one muscle set at a time, but work on several sets together. The effect of this is that other parts of your face are recruited for the exercises – so you are actually getting far more overall benefit. Furthermore, because you are using your fingers to provide resistance, which adds extra weight to the exercise, you'll get better results – much faster.

Generally speaking, most women (and men) find that the areas of the face that need the most help to stay looking good are:

- Cheeks
- Forehead and eyebrows
- Jawline, mouth and laughter lines
- Under chin, neck and jowls

Before starting the natural face-lift routine related to these four areas, please remember these important guidelines:

- Put your mind into the muscles being worked. You'll know that you are doing it right as you'll actually feel all the muscle contractions and, in many cases, you'll see results instantly, as the muscles get pumped up.

- Your fingers are there for resistance, so do remember to use them in that way, rather than to push or pull your skin in any way. It might be helpful to visualize them being like weights or resistance bands that are there to make the exercise stronger – so that you get results faster.

- I'm only giving you *suggested* reps and sets, as we all have such different needs, so just do each exercise until you feel it. These exercises really do work wonders, but only if you actually put the work in and do them.

- Facial exercises are fantastic, but if you aren't looking after your skin by cleansing and moisturizing it properly (see page 154) and by doing other techniques like my facial acupressure (see page 168) and lymphatic drainage (see page 165–6), you'll be missing out on very helpful additions that – all used together – will make a huge difference to your looks.

REWIND PRACTICE – OVER TO YOU
Natural Face-Lift Exercise 1: Cheek Lift

1. Begin by curling the index fingers of both hands into "C" shapes and place them just below your cheekbones on both sides of your face.
2. Push your cheek muscles upward. You'll notice that pushing your cheeks upward causes a bit of scrunching of the skin around your eyes; this is OK, as it is only temporary.
3. Now, holding your cheek muscles upward as best you can, open your mouth into an elongated "O" shape. Very important: after you open your mouth into an elongated "O", check to make sure that you aren't scrunching your eyes up. If you allow your eyes to scrunch, it could make that area worse. Practise in front of a mirror a few times to make sure that you get it right.
4. Hold for a count of 10, remembering that you are meant to be pushing against the resistance of your fingers.
5. Repeat 10 times, relaxing briefly between each time you do it.

Natural Face-Lift Exercise 2:
Forehead/Eyebrow Lift

1. Standing or sitting in front of a mirror to make sure you're not scrunching up your face, begin by finding the natural arch of your eyebrow and place your index fingers right on it.
2. Lift your brows with your fingertips.
3. Now, try to push your eyebrows down against the resistance of your fingertips, and hold for a slow count of five. You should be able to see the result there and then – the reason being that you've signalled to the muscles what you want them to do and they will obey!
4. Repeat 10 times and, if you like, at other points throughout the day, too.

Natural Face-Lift Exercise 3:
Jawline, Mouth and Laughter Lines (Naso-Labial Folds)

1. Ensure you have nice clean hands and then begin by hooking your index fingers inside your mouth, against the insides of your cheeks.
2. Without stretching your skin, make a big smile and then, just using the power of your facial muscles, pull your fingers together. Try to make them touch. They won't, but that's the image you need to have in mind. It's extremely important to make sure you use your fingers as the resistance

mechanism in this exercise – and *not* to pull your mouth wide. This way, you will ensure that the face muscles are doing all the work.

3. Hold the squeeze for a count of 10 and release.
4. Repeat 10 times. You will really feel this one, but, my goodness, it works!

Natural Face-Lift Exercise 4:
Under Chin, Neck and Jowls

1. Put your lower lip up over your upper lip and try to get it as high up as you can, as if you're trying to touch it to your nose.
2. Now gently lean your head back, try to smile and hold for a count of 10. You should really feel the pull in your neck and under your chin.
3. Repeat any time you get the chance throughout the day.

Lymphatic Drainage Facial

Lymphatic drainage is another wonderful technique that has huge benefits for your face. It will relax and rejuvenate your facial and neck muscles, relieve tension and assist in detoxification. In doing so, it will reduce eye puffiness, eye bags, dark circles, wrinkles and fine lines; prevent you from looking so tired; and overall help you to achieve firmer, softer, younger-looking skin. Note that I'm avoiding the term "massage" here and have instead opted to call this approach a "process". This is because the pressure required to achieve proper lymph drainage is so light and delicate that to call it a massage would do it a disservice. As you'll soon discover, applying too much pressure would be completely counterproductive.

First of all, what is "lymph"?

Our lymphatic system is essential to the health and proper functioning of our immune system. It is part of our circulatory system, and as discussed in Chapter 11, it has no pump; instead, it relies on our bodily movement to circulate, through lymph vessels, around the body. Lymph is a clear fluid (its name comes from the Latin *lympha*, meaning water), and it is vital for our health that it circulates freely, as our lymph vessels are crucial in the collection of cellular metabolic waste – and even transport bits of viruses, bacteria and other pathogens away from infected tissue.

Lymph travels to our lymph nodes (sometimes called "glands"), where it is "scanned" and the cells in the lymph node respond rapidly to mount a coordinated and very specific immune response to the pathogen. A really good example of lymph nodes in action is when we have a sore throat and our glands swell under our jaw and in our neck.

Although scientific research in this area is still in its infancy, there seems to be a growing body of evidence that lymphatic drainage really does keep us looking younger. For example, intriguing recent research concluded that impaired function of lymphatic vessels can lead to accumulation of subcutaneous fat, which leads to sagging skin. Furthermore, the study then looked at the way that a particular extract of a pine cone (from Scots Pine, or *Pinus sylvestris*) can strengthen and normalize impaired lymph vessels. The researchers conducted the trial for two months, after which it was noted that sagging skin on the volunteers' neck area was decreased and there was a marked improvement in the skin-sagging around their laughter lines (naso-labial lines) as well as other facial lines, too.

Using Therapeutic Lymph Drainage

Therapeutic lymph drainage gently moves excess lymphatic fluid from your tissues through your lymph channels into your lymph nodes, where it is cleaned and processed before being emptied into blood vessels near your heart, ready to circulate around your body again. This helps to reduce swelling and puffiness, improve immune function and lessen any pain.

It requires a very light touch – just enough to move and lightly stretch your skin – so, as already mentioned, it's best not to think of it as a massage as such. Think of making a circular movement that starts off light and gets even lighter as you approach the lymph node – so up, out and down on either side of the face (which means that your fingers are going in different directions on each side of the face). You are gently "brushing" the fluid, so "less is more". Any deeper pressure would be counterproductive, as it would block the lymph channels. The idea is to help the lymph fluid move "top down"; gravity also helps with this, of course.

The simplified diagram opposite shows the approximate locations of some of the key lymph nodes and their adjoining channels. Please note that this is in no way meant to be a medical representation of the node system as this would require a diagram of much greater complexity. Rather, it is simply to give you an idea of the main areas that we will be focusing on in the lymphatic drainage work that follows: around the ears, the lower part of the face, the back of the head and neck.

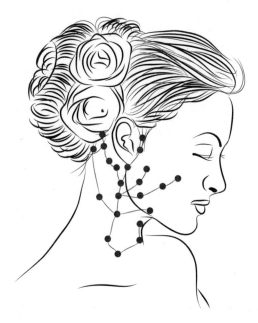

Above: Representation of some of the key lymph nodes and channels in the face and neck.

REWIND PRACTICE – OVER TO YOU
Step-by-Step Lymphatic Drainage Facial

As you follow the steps below, feel free to look back at the diagram above at any time if you feel it helps you maintain an awareness of the approximate location of the nodes. Don't worry about trying to find each specific point though; the artwork is just to give you an overall sense. Although we are mainly working to enhance the youthfulness of the face, the exercise will start at base of the neck in order to clear the channels and allow fluid to drain more easily during the rest of the steps.

1. Place the first three fingertips of both hands slightly above the inside bony edges of your collarbones (clavicles), and make smooth, very light outward circles on your skin. Think about just moving the skin – definitely not the muscle beneath it. Do this for approximately a minute.
2. Slowly move up your neck to the area in front of your ears, gently circling at each point you choose along the way for a minute – in order to clear the channels of the neck.
3. Next, lift your hands, place the same three fingers of each hand under either side of your chin, and slowly and gently make small outward

circles here. Visualize that you are very lightly "encouraging" the lymph under your chin to move down into your neck nodes.

4. Now place your fingers just under your ears and lightly stroke them along the line of the jaw, to the chin, and down to just above the inner edge of the collarbones. Lift your hands back up to just under your ears and repeat this downward stroking movement for approximately a minute.

5. Next, place your fingers at the base of your skull, on the back of your head, and stroke your fingers diagonally downwards and around your neck to arrive just above the inner edge of your collarbones. Continue to repeat this gentle downward stoking for approximately a minute.

6. Now bring your hands to either side of your chin and make small, gentle outward circular movements for approximately a minute, before moving your hands up slightly to make the same circular movement midway between your chin and each ear – all the time remembering to keep your touch feather-light. Then move your fingers up to make the same small circles just in front of the ears for a minute, then on your temples and finally on the middle of either side of the forehead.

7. Repeat Step 5.

8. This time gently stroke your fingertips from your temples, down the sides of your face, to your jawline, under your jaw and down to just above the clavicular nodes – to encourage the downward flow of the lymph. Continue this for approximately one minute.

9. Lastly, do three downward routes with your hands: long, medium and short. For the first, start with your fingers at the base of the skull, on the back of your head, give your skin a gentle stretch outward and downward and then slowly move your hands around the sides of your neck and down to the inner edge of your collarbones, stopping at points along the way to give the skin another gentle stretch for a few seconds each time. Next, do the same incremental stretching process, but this time starting at the front of the ears and working down the sides of the neck to just above the collarbones. And finally do the same again, this time starting just under the centre of the jaw and working down to your collarbones.

Contraindications for Lymph Work

The type of therapeutic lymphatic drainage that you have just learned is used in many settings, including by physiotherapists to assist fluid movement when people have had lymph nodes removed, so it it's very safe. It's important to know that it's not just a treatment to help you look more vibrant; it can also be used to address blunt-force traumas and after facial surgery. However, this requires advanced training.

As it is such an effective and powerful therapy, there are several contraindications to be aware of, so do *not* perform lymphatic drainage if you have:

- An active infection such as sinusitis, strep throat, a tooth abscess or any skin infection
- Head and neck cancers
- Idiopathic facial swelling

Acupressure for a Natural Face-Lift

Another natural facial exercise technique that you might like to try as an alternative to either the four-part Face-Lift Routine or the Lymphatic Drainage Facial is the Acupressure Facial Routine on the page overleaf. Simply expressed, acupressure is an ancient Chinese healing practice that works on the same principle as acupuncture, but using your own fingers instead of needles. During a treatment, pressure is applied to the energy channels in your body known as meridians to allow energy (or *chi*) to flow more smoothly and easily throughout your body. In Traditional Chinese Medicine (TCM) it is thought that disease occurs at points where *chi* stagnates. Acupressure stimulates and clears these points, resulting in restored health, by applying pressure to them while rubbing in circular motions.

The facial acupressure regime that you'll learn in a moment is one that you can do safely at home to delay signs of ageing, tighten up and tone your face and – because acupressure works with your body's meridians – also help to balance and tone other bodily organs.

You may notice when you begin the treatment that some of the points feel a little tender. In TCM, this is considered a good thing as it means you have a chance to move and clear the energy (or *chi*) that is stuck at that point. So, keep at it. Just be sure not to overdo it. Listen to your body at all times. A slight tenderness is a good thing; actual pain is not. Breathe deeply during your treatment session and focus your mind on each point.

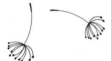

REWIND PRACTICE – OVER TO YOU
Step-by-Step Facial Acupressure Routine

Here follows the five-step Facial Acupressure Routine that I do every night. I find it works incredibly well, and I notice a difference if I neglect to do it for a while. It could be done at any time of day, but it is best to do it either first thing in the morning or last thing at night.

See the diagram opposite for the location of each energy point included in the routine, noting that almost all points in this routine can be worked on in pairs – one on each side of the face.

Use medium pressure on each point, moving your fingers in small circles (you can make inward or outward circles depending on what's easiest for you in each location, and what feels natural), and stimulate each point for approximately 10 seconds before moving on to the next point.

Start by just using your fingers to apply the pressure to each point. Once you become comfortable with the routine, you might want to experiment with applying pressure in different ways to see if it yields different results. For example, you could choose to use your knuckle.

Point 1 Jingming: Located on the inside edge of each eye. This is particularly helpful for sore, tired eyes and as a preventative against eye problems.

Point 2 Zanzhu: Located on the inside end of each eyebrow. This is particularly good to help with frontal headaches, sore, tired eyes and sinus pain, and as a preventative against eye problems.

Point 3 Taiyang: Located on the temples to the side of each eye. This is particularly good to help ease either one or two-sided headaches, to calm the mind, and for eye problems.

Point 4 Yingxiang: Located next to each nostril. This is particularly good to help prevent and treat nasal congestion, sinusitis and rhinitis.

Point 5 Renzhong: Located under your nose, on the midline. Using your knuckle or the tip of your middle or index finger to press this point draws energy up to your head and helps your nasal passages adjust to weather changes. It can also be used as a revival point after fainting or shock and has been successfully used to resuscitate wounded soldiers who have gone into shock and has therefore saved many lives. Personnel in the US Army are undergoing training to learn more acupuncture techniques like this.

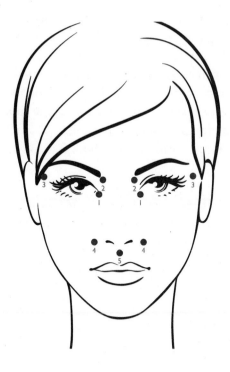

Above: Some of the key acupressure points on the face.

When to Do the Natural Face-Lift Routine, Lymphatic Drainage Facial and Facial Acupressure Routine

We're all different, so I expect that as you experiment with the various techniques just outlined, you are likely to develop preferences for some over others. However, I just wanted to remind you in case you decide to incorporate all three into your Rewind Journey that, as I mentioned at the start of this chapter, the three step-by-step exercises just presented are *not* meant to be done one after the other. Through a lot of trial and error over the years, I have worked out that it is best to do:

- Lymphatic Drainage Facial in the morning
- Natural Facelift Routine any time throughout the day
- Facial Acupressure Routine at night

It's definitely best to avoid doing the lymphatic drainage and acupressure exercises close together as the pressure needed to stimulate the acupoints would temporarily squash the lymph channels, meaning they wouldn't be able to drain fully. Don't worry – they'd soon spring back, but I'm all for an easy life so we might as well be as efficient as possible and avoid one treatment cancelling out the effects of the other!

Whichever ones you choose to do at whatever times, each process is extremely powerful in its own right, so I do urge you to incorporate the ones you feel you get the most from into your life as much as you can so that you start seeing results as soon as possible. Above all else, have fun with them, as that in itself will help you both feel and look younger!

Your Youthful Skin Mindset Moving Forward:

Now that you've come to the end of this chapter, take a little time to think about its content and come up with a specific, positive, present-tense Mindset Phrase of your own for the topic in hand, focusing on the information that has resonated most with you from the chapter.

CHAPTER 14
LUSCIOUS LOCKS

*" I commit to using the natural tips in this chapter
to enhance my beautiful hair by making it more
luscious, healthy and youthful. "*

I adore folk remedies as I find the stories behind how they came about fascinating. As we know, they are often disparaged and dismissed by mainstream healthcare practitioners and, in some cases, quite rightly of course. However, the more I research what is actually behind some of them, the more I realize how many of these traditions – handed down from mother to daughter – have immense value. In this chapter you'll learn how to use tried-and-tested home remedies based on ancient folk remedies to get thicker, glossier, younger-looking hair – quickly.

I lost a lot of hair when I became very ill, and then lost even more when I was advised to take methotrexate (MTX) – a chemotherapy drug used in rheumatoid arthritis at low dose. (In leukaemia treatment it is used at a higher dose – but for shorter duration.) I took MTX for five years in total – with very unpleasant results. One of the most noticeable side effects was severe hair loss. I went on a serious quest to figure out what steps I could take to regrow my hair as fast as possible – focused on finding options that were both *scientifically* proven to work and safe to use alongside my medications. And the result is that I ended up discovering an array of natural ways to enhance hair growth and health!

Even if you're not dealing with hair loss from medication, it's not uncommon for us to experience hair thinning and hair loss as we get older. In fact, by the age of 50, about 50 per cent of women and 85 per cent of men are believed to have experienced some degree of hair loss. As a result of this, there are a multitude of hair-loss prevention products on the market. Unfortunately, however, these generally tend to be chemically-based and contain substances that are known hormone disruptors, such as formaldehyde, parabens, oxybenzones, sodium lauryl (ether) sulphate (SLS, SLES) etc. I therefore personally choose to avoid these, as substantial evidence shows that they are harmful to health.

Instead, I call on my array of effective home remedies. On the pages that follow you will find my three favourite of these for you to try as part of your Rewind Journey. Although the onion one in particular may seem a little unusual at first, I use these every time I wash my hair and am always amazed at how vibrant they leave my locks looking, so I hope you experience the same positive results.

Remember that it's wise when using any remedies for the first time to do a patch test before using the product for real. Do this by rubbing a drop of it behind your ear and waiting for 24 hours to see for any reaction.

The Growth-Enhancing Power of Rosemary Oil

Rosemary essential oil has been shown as an effective treatment for both hair loss and baldness associated with an excess of dihydrotestosterone (DHT), a testosterone by-product that causes male pattern baldness and also some baldness in women (as we produce testosterone too). Among the research backing up its efficacy is a 2013 study of mice, in which testosterone-related hair loss was reversed when treated with rosemary oil. It turns out that the rosemary oil inhibits DHT from binding to hormone receptors that enable it to attack the hair follicles. In a 2015 study, people with DHT-related hair loss were given either rosemary oil or minoxidil (a conventional hair-regrowth treatment) for six months. Both groups saw significant increases in hair growth, but the group using the rosemary oil experienced more than the minoxidil group. Furthermore, the rosemary oil didn't cause any of the side effects of minoxidil. A 2017 study also demonstrated that rosemary oil kills some fungi and bacteria, so if hair loss is due to an infection or unhealthy scalp, rosemary oil might help.

Rosemary oil has even been shown to be of benefit to people with *Alopecia areata*, an autoimmune disorder that causes bald patches. In a study, 44 per cent of participants with this distressing condition improved with the use of rosemary over seven months, compared to just 15 per cent who received no treatment. See the "Rewind Practice" opposite for how to make a gentle anti-ageing shampoo using this amazing essential oil.

REWIND PRACTICE – OVER TO YOU
Making a Rosemary Shampoo

To make a hair-enhancing rosemary shampoo that would be suitable for everyday use, if desired, simply:

1. Add 10–12 drops of organic rosemary essential oil to a bottle of organic baby shampoo bought at any supermarket or health store, and mix well.
2. Then apply the rosemary blend to your hair as you would any ordinary shampoo, lather it up and let it sit for two minutes before washing it off.

There is some evidence to show that the longer the oil is in contact with your scalp, the more effective it is, so if you'd like to make an overnight treatment for occasional use too, you can do this by adding just a couple of drops of the rosemary oil to a tablespoon of carrier oil; I love coconut oil for its super-conditioning effect, as well as its lovely tropical scent, although you need to melt it before use as it is solid at room temperature.

1. Just blend this thoroughly, apply it to your scalp – and right through to the ends of your hair if you want to take advantage of the super-conditioning effects – before you go to bed. Be sure to put a towel on your pillow so the oil doesn't make a mess!
2. The next morning, add a little water to your homemade shampoo and lather it up so that it's extra-foamy. Then add this to your hair to break down the oil without stripping your hair of the moisturizing treatment.
3. Finally, just wash your shampoo out as normal. Just be aware that you might need to "rinse and repeat", as coconut oil is quite a heavy oil so takes a bit of getting rid of! But I promise the results are worth it!

Remember: It's always a good idea to do a small patch test, as explained on the page opposite, before using a new remedy more widely.

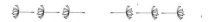

The Unexpected Power of Onion Juice

It may initially sound odd, but, believe it or not, onion juice has been used for centuries to alleviate hair loss that we now know is related to DHT, and it's also been shown to be effective for the regrowth of hair in people with *Alopecia areata*. As an extra bonus, it conditions hair beautifully, too. A 2002 study, the results of which were published in the *Journal of Dermatology*, showed that hair growth commenced after just two weeks of applying onion juice twice daily to the scalp of people with alopecia. Almost 74 per cent of the participants had some hair regrowth after four weeks, and about 87 per cent had some after six weeks.

Although we don't know precisely how onion juice acts to regrow hair, it is thought that nutrients in the juice, including bio-available sulphur, nourish the hair follicles, which increases volume and shine – explaining the conditioning aspect. This extra nourishment also enhances hair strength, reducing breakages and thinning. Plus, active components in the juice are believed to have the capacity to lengthen the growing phase of the hair, which means your hair will remain within its follicle longer before it sheds, resulting in longer hair if you want it.

REWIND PRACTICE – OVER TO YOU
Making an Onion Juice Wonder Remedy

You should be able to buy onion juice online these days, but if you'd like to make an onion juice tonic of your own that you can use as a wonderful hair conditioner or hair-restorer, just follow these steps:

1. Peel about four onions and chop them into small pieces.
2. Extract the juice out of the onion by either squeezing it or using a juicer. Alternatively, blend the onion pieces into a paste, place the paste in a cheesecloth and squeeze all the juice out.
3. If you would like to improve the odour of the juice, add a few drops of an essential oil such as peppermint, lavender or rosemary.
4. Then simply massage the juice into your scalp twice a day – morning and night – and leave it to dry in each time. Once it has dried, there really isn't an "oniony" smell, so there's no need to worry about that.

Note: Even if you can *eat* onion without any problem, it's advised to do a patch test behind your ear, as advised on page 172, before applying this remedy to your scalp as it is still possible that your *skin* might react to it.

The Power of Apple Cider Vinegar (ACV)

I use an apple cider vinegar rinse when I wash my hair, as it helps to maintain glossy hair, keeps your scalp clear and stops any itching. Personally, I find that it also allows my hair to reflect light more, which gives it even more of a sheen than I might normally get. These benefits are as a result of the natural acidity of the liquid, which helps to smooth the hair cuticles, enabling knots and tangles to slip right out so that frizz and breakages are dramatically reduced.

Some dermatologists report that the anti-inflammatory and antimicrobial properties of apple cider vinegar may combat the yeast and irritation that lead to the build-up of dead skin cells, flakes and itching, all of which can compromise optimal hair growth and condition.

  REWIND PRACTICE – OVER TO YOU
Making a Shine-Enhancing ACV Rinse

To make an apple cider vinegar blend that you can use as often as you want as a post-shampoo conditioning rinse, simply follow the steps below. I've found that the vinegary smell of the ACV wears off as soon as your hair dries, but if you feel concerned, by all means add a few drops of either rosemary or lavender essential oil to the blend.

1. Mix 4 tablespoons of apple cider vinegar with 500ml (17fl oz / 2 cups) of cool water in a bottle and stir well.
2. After washing your hair with your homemade rosemary shampoo (see page 173), or any other gentle shampoo of your choice (an organic baby shampoo can be nice), thoroughly rinse the shampoo out.
3. Then follow this up with the apple cider vinegar rinse. To use it, just gently tilt your head back and pour it over your entire scalp, making sure you don't get any in your eyes.
4. There's no need to wash it out as it is a conditioning rinse – just allow your hair to dry and any vinegary smell will dissipate.

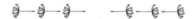

Tips to Keep Your Hair in Tip-Top Shape

• Ditch the cotton: Avoid using a cotton towel to dry your hair as cotton fibres and loops get caught on your hair, ripping open the cuticles and exacerbating frizz. I use a microfibre fabric instead, which provides a smooth surface to absorb the water quickly.

• Lose the heat: It's best to minimize how much you expose your hair to heat, whether from hairdryers, tongs, straighteners or whatever else, as, despite what the manufacturers of these products may claim, there's nothing that deconditions hair faster. Simply let your hair dry naturally instead whenever possible or, if you feel you absolutely have to style your hair with heat, then use the lowest settings possible.

Your Luscious Locks Mindset Moving Forward:
Now that you've come to the end of this chapter, take a little time to think about its content and come up with a specific, positive, present-tense Mindset Phrase of your own for the topic in hand, focusing on the information that has resonated most with you from the chapter.

CHAPTER 15
NATURAL HORMONAL BALANCE

66 *Perfectly balanced hormones are my birthright. I choose activities that will rewind my body clock and promote hormonal wellbeing.* 99

Hormonal imbalances affect both men and women. In men, the primary age-related disruption centres around decreasing levels of two hormones: HGH (see Chapter 12) and testosterone. This can lead to a lack of motivation, poorer muscle-to-fat ratio, depleted libido and more. However, thankfully, it can be prevented with the lifestyle approaches in this book and also via natural hormone replacement if a boost is required.

Women are rather more complicated. We, too, have falling levels of HGH and testosterone (albeit in much smaller amounts than men). Plus, as we approach the menopause (in a phase known as the peri-menopause), we start noticing symptoms, such as hot flushes (flashes), mood swings, difficulty sleeping, weight gain (especially around the middle), and reduced sexual desire – all of which can make us feel old before our time.

However, you mustn't feel that you are doomed to an uncomfortable menopause. In fact, research shows that the very lifestyle changes in this book can help to prevent menopause symptoms. Women who eat mainly plant-based diets, exercise consistently and have stress-management strategies (such as following a meditation practice and healthy social lives etc.), tend to have less extreme symptoms. And it is fascinating to note the absence of the word "menopause" among women in rural Japan, Singapore and among the Mayans in Mexico, as they don't have the same uncomfortable symptoms that we have in industrialized nations.

Redressing the Balance

I would estimate that 90 per cent of the women I see in my complementary health practice have hormonal imbalance as a major contributing factor in the health issues they are experiencing. Happily, however, there are steps that can be taken at any age to naturally balance our hormone levels – which will, in turn, help us to both look and feel younger, with enhanced energy, libido and enthusiasm for life.

The first ports of call when it comes to balancing our hormones, and therefore generally enhancing youthful vibrancy, have already been covered elsewhere in this book, such as stress resilience strategies including meditation (see Chapter 5), nutrition (see Chapter 6), exercise (see Chapter 12), and sociability (see the next chapter).

In this chapter, we're therefore going to look at a few other key areas: firstly substances that we're regularly exposed to that can put our hormones off balance in the *first* place – known as "hormone disruptors" – so that we can reduce our exposure to them; and then I'll give you my choice of top natural remedies that have been used in various cultures for thousands of years to keep women's hormonal systems vibrant and functioning well. The remedies I cover will help you to lose that "blah" feeling hormonal imbalance can cause, and to really get your mojo back on all levels.

Avoid Hormone Disruptors

One of the most fundamental steps to take when looking at how to achieve optimal hormonal balance is to think about ways to avoid environmental toxins. It is now well known, for example, that substances such as Bisphenol A (BPA) and phthalates found in plastics, and also parabens, which are commonly found in shampoos, body washes and the like, can severely disrupt our hormonal systems.

When functioning well, our endocrine (hormonal) system releases hormones that send signals to various tissues telling them what to do. However, when chemicals from the outside that have a similar molecular shape to our *own* hormones – called "xenoestrogens", deriving from the Greek *xeno*, meaning foreign – enter our bodies, they have the ability to mimic the activity of our hormones, thus disrupting the normal functioning of our endocrine system. This is highly detrimental to hormone-sensitive organs such as the uterus, endometrium (the membrane lining the uterus), the prostate and testes in men, and the neurological systems, immune systems and breast tissue in both genders.

Our bodies normally regulate the amount of oestrogen that we need through intricate biochemical pathways. However, when xenoestrogens (such as BPA or phthalates) enter the body, they increase the amount of total oestrogen, resulting in a phenomenon called oestrogen dominance. And as xenoestrogens aren't water-soluble (meaning we can't pee them out), our bodies instead store a build-up of them in fat cells, which has the capacity to contribute to the development of many problems, including obesity, infertility, acne, endometriosis, miscarriages and type 2 diabetes.

Unfortunately, the long list of products containing hormone-disrupting compounds, such as xenoestrogen, is growing daily, as greater numbers of chemical compounds are being created and finding their way into usage in products that we use in daily life; estimates vary as to how many hormone-disrupting compounds we are exposed to every day. This is bad enough in itself, but the even bigger problem is that the effect of them in *combination* is likely to be exponentially magnified.

Below are some everyday things to avoid as much as possible, as they are among the worst hormone-disruptor sources:

- The combined oral contraceptive pill.
- Make-up, sunscreen and nail polish that contain parabens or benzophenone; you can now get organic ones that are safe.
- Plastic products, such as lunchboxes, water bottles, food-wrap and sandwich bags (and, strangely enough, also till receipts); most companies now tend to state if their products are BPA-free as so many people are aware of the dangers these days – so do read the labels.
- Household cleaning products containing chemicals called alkylphenol ethoxylates. These are banned in the EU but still in use in the US and are not necessarily listed on products, so it's best to use organic products instead. There's also a risk that clothes and fabrics imported from countries that still ubiquitously use this chemical are contaminated, so it's advised to wash all new clothes before wearing them.
- Flame-retardant fabrics or substances (we are only just beginning to understand just how dangerous these substances are).

And below are some other suggested changes for you to consider in order to limit your exposure to harmful hormone disruptors:

- Eat organic food wherever possible as these foods won't be sprayed with toxic pesticides, fungicides, bactericides or insecticides. (See the "Dirty Dozen" on page 76 for a list of the most chemically contaminated foods.)

- If you can't get organic food, then wash all fruit and vegetables as thoroughly as possible before eating.
- Cut all dairy out of your diet.
- Choose and use organic beauty products.
- Avoid storing or heating food in plastic containers, or eating from them. Use alternatives such as glass or ceramic instead.
- Choose unbleached sanitary products, teabags and bedclothes; they will generally be labelled as such.
- Always air any dry-cleaned clothes before storing or wearing them as the chemicals used to clean them are considered "probable carcinogens" by the USA's Environmental Protection Agency (EPA).
- Avoid spending too much time at photocopiers, as they emit high levels of toxic particulates.

Herbs for Enhancing Vitality and Healthy Longevity

The herbs and other natural remedies that follow have been used by women for millennia in cultures around the world to help balance hormones in different ways. However, as with all herbs, it is vital to carefully check all labels and/or check with your health practitioner if in any doubt as to whether they are suitable for you and, if so, how to use them. Formulations vary, and the strength or dosage of herbs in any preparation may differ. Also be sure to check for any allergies.

Most of the remedies in the pages that follow are available in capsule form unless otherwise stated. You'll notice that many of them have particular aphrodisiac qualities. Given that a loss of interest in sex and decreased sexual enjoyment as we get older can be due to *hormonal* imbalance, using such remedies to redress this imbalance can really enhance natural confidence, energy and outlook as well as restoring libido, making us feel overall much younger and more vibrant.

Ashwagandha

Ashwagandha is one of the most important herbs in Ayurvedic medicine (India's age-old holistic healing system). Used over thousands of years, it has been shown to reduce stress hormones (including cortisol), which can disrupt endocrine function, increase deposits of fat around the midriff and contribute toward premature ageing. Ashwagandha also stimulates blood flow to female reproductive organs, therefore increasing sensitivity and arousal. This makes it a particularly popular choice among women who wish to derive more sexual pleasure and/or regain lost sex drive. Women going through the menopause also find that it helps to reduce anxiety, depression and hot flushes (flashes). Plus the herb is a powerful ally in the fight against chronic inflammation, truly making it one of the most important pieces of the natural anti-ageing jigsaw.

It comes in loose herb, tea and capsule form, and can be bought at any health food store or online. I have found better and more potent varieties from Ayurvedic practitioners though; you can find many listed on The Complementary Medical Association's website (The-CMA.org.uk).

Maca

This root, also known as "Peruvian ginseng", has been used for thousands of years by the native people of the Andes to address issues such as infertility, hot flushes (flashes), sexual dysfunction, sleep disruptions and even night sweats associated with the menopause. As maca is loaded with phytonutrients and zinc, it is a commonly used aphrodisiac and libido stimulant; women who use maca commonly report greater sexual desire and improved sexual satisfaction.

I find that maca is something of an acquired taste, so it is best to start with a small dose. I've worked up to taking about a flat tablespoon per day in my smoothies. Brands do differ though, so if you don't like the first one you try, shop around a bit to see if you can find one that you prefer.

Avena Sativa

This is the Latin name for common oats, which have been used for aeons in all sorts of contexts to provide fast energy; it's one of the reasons they are fed to racehorses (among other high-energy feeds). Scientific research now shows that *avena sativa* is an effective libido enhancer, too, as well as helping to alleviate menstrual cramps. This is because it both improves blood flow and stimulates the central nervous system. It is also believed by researchers to free "bound testosterone" to make it more available throughout the body, which is an essential hormone for sexual desire in both men and women. You can buy it as liquid or in capsule form.

Catuaba Bark

Traditionally used by the Tupi Indians of Brazil, this bark, found mainly as a capsule preparation, is particularly known as a libido enhancer as it contains yohimbine, which stimulates the central nervous system, therefore enhancing both energy and mood. Caution is advised with this, however, as it can cause heart-racing sensations in some people. It's therefore best to consult with a qualified herbalist to check its suitability for you.

Damiana

This time-honoured herb has been used over millennia, including by Mayans, to improve sexual interest and desire. Recent research shows that it is a superb sexual "pick-me-up" for both men and women. Several other studies show that a preparation containing damiana, ginseng and ginkgo increased sexual satisfaction in women. And two to three cups of damiana tea per week can make menopausal symptoms disappear for many women.

Epimedium

This herb, sometimes known as "horny goat weed", can help with loss of libido (as suggested by its nickname) but also has outstanding menopause-relieving effects. It has been found to act similarly to testosterone and is far more effective for some people than many current drug therapies, but without the side effects.

Ginseng

Ginseng is another herb that has potent pro-sexual powers. Although it has traditionally been used for millennia throughout Ancient China by men to improve energy and erections, recent research has shown that menopausal women taking ginseng felt aroused more easily and reported overall improvements in their sex lives. Be aware, however, that ginseng can cause headaches, insomnia and palpitations in sensitive people. See Chapter 10 (pages 122–4) on adaptogenic herbs for more about the different types of Ginseng and their varying health and wellness benefits.

Muira Puama

This herb, also known as "potency wood", works to calm the nerves, relieve anxiety, fight fatigue, improve cognitive function and promote a healthy stress response, as well as increasing blood flow to the pelvic area. Many women who regularly take *Muira puama* report increased sexual desire, more satisfying intercourse and more intense orgasms. In trials it has also been shown to improve bone density – good for osteoporosis sufferers.

Rhodiola

As we know from Chapter 8, rhodiola – sometimes known as "golden root" – is an adaptogen, which means it can balance mind, mood and body, helping to manage your stress responses (see also page 123). Aside from these adaptogenic effects, rhodiola also powerfully boosts sexual response, primarily by improving energy levels in a sustainable way, unlike caffeine or other stimulants.

Suma

Sometimes referred to as "South American ginseng", this herb has been traditionally used to improve mood and stimulate sexual desire. It has been shown in research to increase levels of oestradiol 17 beta, which is a powerful sex hormone necessary for well-balanced hormone levels and reproductive health.

Shilajit

Shilajit alleviates anxiety, lifts mood and stimulates overall health. It has been used for many thousands of years in both traditional Indian and Chinese medicine. The Chinese consider it a tonic that aids physical energy and sexual drive. Formed from organic compressed plant material from the Himalayas, it is packed with nutrients, amino acids and antioxidants, and its fulvic acid passes easily across the intestinal barrier, which improves healthy antioxidant availability.

Shilajit tastes bitter, so it's wise to build up your tolerance. I started taking a quarter of a teaspoon per day at first and can only tolerate about half a teaspoon at best – but I do notice a difference in my energy levels.

Tongcat Ali

This herb, used by women in Southeast Asia who wish to stimulate their libido and erogenous sensitivity, is often thought of as the greatest aphrodisiac known to humankind. As well as having the power to improve all aspects of our sexual response, it can boost energy levels, improve cognitive function and enhance resilience by regulating our responses to stress. Tongcat ali also boosts testosterone levels, promoting all-round optimal hormonal balance.

Tribulus Testris

Used for many hundreds of years in both Chinese and Indian cultures, *Tribulus testris* has a long-held reputation as an aphrodisiac. A lot of women who use the herb experience increased arousal, better sexual satisfaction and improved health of the reproductive system. It also has a variety of other health benefits, including the ability to encourage the body to use hormones more efficiently, to reduce blood sugar and to lower cholesterol levels.

REWIND PRACTICE – OVER TO YOU
Get Your Hormones Tested

If you're considering using any of the herbs or supplements just discussed to balance your hormones, it can be a good idea to first have your hormone levels checked by a trusted healthcare professional if possible.

The issue, however, is that most hormonal imbalances that women in particular experience are subtle, including tiredness, weight gain, thinning hair and so on – and most doctors aren't trained to recognize that symptoms like this together may indicate hormonal imbalance. You might therefore struggle to get tests or even to get a doctor to recognize that you have a problem. Patients of mine have been told in the past that they should just expect all these symptoms at this time of life as that's "just what happens to women". This doesn't sit well with me. And for this reason I have curated an array of test providers on my website, JayneyGoddard.org, to help you navigate where it might be possible to have such tests done if you would like them.

It is very useful to know your own hormonal status, as you will then be in a position to better understand which natural remedies are likely to be best for you as an individual. Your status is likely to vary at different times, so it's best to get tested approximately every year if you are in balance, or more frequently if you are experiencing uncomfortable symptoms.

Once you have better hormonal balance, hopefully achieved by implementing many of the lifestyle approaches in this book, including using some of the herbs in this chapter, you can reduce the frequency of testing. I should point out though that I don't recommend testing for its own sake. It should only be done when you feel that there is a real reason for it. Otherwise, it can be a waste of your time and money.

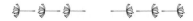

Your Hormonal Balance Mindset Moving Forward:
Now that you've come to the end of this chapter, take a little time to think about its content and come up with a specific, positive, present-tense Mindset Phrase of your own for the topic in hand, focusing on the information that has resonated most with you from the chapter.

CHAPTER 16

THE POWER OF RELATIONSHIPS AND SOCIABILITY

> **❝** *I value and cultivate good close friendships and thrive on the youth-promoting power of socializing and having fun with friends, knowing that we are all contributing to each other's wellbeing.* **❞**

If I had to put my finger on one lifestyle factor above all others that leads to the greatest gains in terms of both a longer lifespan *and* health-span, I would have to choose "sociability" – that is to say the capacity to be sociable and build good relationships with other people. Across all the research on the subject, this has been proven time and again to be the easiest factor to associate with healthy longevity.

No one knows exactly why "sociability" is so important to wellbeing and enhancement of health-span, as there are so many factors associated with it. However, studies in this area of research show that having an active, fulfilling social life can add well over nine healthy years to one's life.

The physical aspects of life such as diet and exercise would seem to be the most *logical* predictors of longevity and, of course, they are extremely important. However, close relationships with your most reliable friends – the people you can call on a bad day and who you know will always be there for you – also contribute hugely to your healthy longevity, maybe more than you might realize.

Interestingly, we also get a huge health-span boost from our interactions with the people we see on a much more casual but regular basis – whether it be your postman, the barista in your local coffee shop, your hairdresser – and so the list continues. Each of these people provide opportunities for all-important face-to-face anti-ageing interactions.

Cultivating a Sociability Mindset

One of the most effective ways of tapping into the incredible anti-ageing power of sociability is to approach relationships with a mindset of:

- What can I do for others?
- How can I make a difference in peoples' lives?
- What random act of kindness can I do today?

Coming from a mindset of unconditional kindness impacts you deeply – mentally, emotionally, physically and spiritually. This is because when we are able to embrace feel-good emotions, our thinking becomes much more creative, integrative, flexible, and we are so much more open to information. And the added bonus is that the benefits of acts and interactions of kindness and compassion touch *everybody*: the giver, the receiver and even witnesses. In fact, even just reading about kindness can have a positive effect on our holistic health.

The Ripple Effect of Loving Kindness

I love the idea that a simple act of kindness has this incredible "ripple effect" and just one small act can have a huge impact on so many others – the compassion spreading out and positively affecting people we know, strangers in our immediate vicinity and then beyond that, into the wider world. As I write this, I'm reminded of the Loving Kindness, or Metta, Meditation technique that I explained on page 56, so do feel free to turn to this earlier chapter to follow this technique at any time to get more into the practice of a kind and loving mindset.

The Anti-Ageing Effects of Compassion and Kindness

Most of us innately sense that living a life filled with love, compassion and social support is likely to have health and wellbeing benefits, and scientific research now bears this out. You might think that it would be tough to study compassion scientifically, yet it is actually one of the fastest growing areas of research in the "positive psychology" arena. I was surprised to learn that it is currently such a hot research topic – particularly in the field of nursing, although increasingly in other conventional medical areas, too.

What follows is a collection of just some of the research that speaks deeply to the effects of love, kindness, compassion and altruism on us all.

A piece of research that I like to call the "Bunny Love Study" (but which is actually called "Social environment as a factor in diet-induced atherosclerosis" – rather more of a mouthful!) is just one brilliant illustration of how receiving acts of kindness actually impacts physical health. In the late 1970s, researchers at Georgia Tech (Georgia Institute of Technology) were studying the effects of a diet high in fat and cholesterol among rabbits. During the study, a rather strange anomaly became apparent: One subgroup of rabbits had 60 per cent less atherosclerosis than the group as a whole, even though they were all eating exactly the same diet. Nobody could figure out why this was, until it emerged that the lab assistant who fed and cared for this particular group of rabbits took them out of their cages, petted them and talked to them before feeding. The study was repeated twice with the same results and was reported in the esteemed journal *Science* in 1980.

Obviously, these findings were gained from animals. However, studies on humans have also proven just how important it is for our health and longevity to live in a loving, nurturing environment, where positive thoughts are likely to flourish. For example, in the 1990s, a group of researchers in the USA revisited an earlier well-known study that had been conducted among nuns who had written short personal essays about

Rewind Insight: It has been shown that the world's longest-lived people reside in what are called the world's "Blue Zones" – a term that was coined by Dan Buettner, a well-respected longevity researcher and author. The original Blue Zones are Okinawa, Japan; Ikaria, Greece; Ogliastra Region, Sardinia; Loma Linda, USA; and the Nicoya Peninsula, Costa Rica. All these places have an extraordinarily high level of super-centenarians – people who live to be older than 100. The really interesting thing about these groups is that while they have different lifestyles in each location, they also have common factors in that they eat healthily – with plant-based foods (and lots of legumes) making up the majority, or entirety, of their diet; they don't smoke; they are moderately and consistently active; and, the strongest common denominator of all, they have both close friendships and robust family ties.

their lives as part of a linguistic study. The results, published in the *Journal of Personality and Social Psychology* in 2001, revealed that the nuns who had expressed the highest number of positive emotions about their life circumstances lived 10 years longer and were also somewhat protected from Alzheimer's disease.

REWIND PRACTICE – OVER TO YOU
Cultivate Unconditional Kindness

To put the notion of more loving kindness into action in everyday life, have a think about what you can do to help someone today. Then plan some other random acts of kindness, too. Here are some ideas to get you started:

- Volunteer at a homeless shelter.
- Sign up for a fundraising walk, run or other event in aid of a good cause.
- Help at an animal rescue centre.
- Hold a fundraiser for a cause close to either your own heart or the heart of someone else you know.
- Pick up litter on the beach or in a local park.
- Let someone go in front of you in a queue.
- Pay a stranger a compliment.
- Make dinner for a friend or family member in need.
- Offer to buy a cinema ticket for the person behind you in the queue.
- Pay for someone's meal at a restaurant.
- Donate Christmas gifts to an orphanage or to a collection point.
- Donate to a charity.
- Hold doors open for people.
- Thank a teacher with a gift.
- Donate your clean old clothes to charity.
- Babysit for free – ideal for new parents who haven't had the time or opportunity to get out.
- Plant a tree – plant anything!
- Do a favour without asking for anything in return.
- Offer to take a new neighbour on a tour of your area.

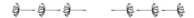

The Positive Power of Selflessness: Helper's High!

Selflessness and altruism are other key social qualities that can help lead to both long-term health and happiness. In fact, a research study published in the journal *Health Psychology* in 2012 showed that a group of retired people over the age of 65 who had volunteered to help others had significantly higher levels of life satisfaction and will to live than control groups of a similar age and background. They also had far fewer symptoms of anxiety, depression and somatisation, which is what used to be called "psychosomatic" illness before the term became stigmatized due to many patients being dismissed with statements like "It's all in your head."

Now, study after study shows that altruistic behaviour in adults is associated with enhanced levels of wellbeing, morale, self-esteem and other positive feelings. In fact, a meta-analysis of studies funded through the Institute for Research on Unlimited Love, and headed by Stephen G. Post, PhD, a professor of bioethics at Case Western Reserve University School of Medicine, showed that two thirds of people who helped others reported distinct positive sensations associated with helping:

- 50 per cent reported a "high" feeling
- 43 per cent felt stronger and more energetic
- 28 per cent felt warm
- 22 per cent felt calmer and less depressed
- 21 per cent felt greater self-worth
- 13 per cent experienced fewer aches and pains

In another study by Field et al. in 1997, older adults massaging infants were shown to have measurably lower levels of stress hormones, including salivary cortisol and plasma norepinephrine and epinephrine. And if these are reduced, so too can chronic inflammation be reduced, with a dramatic impact on anti-ageing.

Even just watching or *thinking* about love, kindness and compassion in action has now been shown to have the capacity to make you physically and emotionally more resilient. In a study undertaken at Harvard in 1987 and published in the journal *Psychology and Health* in 1988, some students were asked to watch a film about Mother Teresa's good work, while others were given the task of "dwelling on love". It was found after the tasks were completed that there was a significant increase in salivary immunoglobin A (the main specific immune defence mechanism in saliva) in both the group *watching* something loving and *thinking about* something loving!

The Effects of Love vs Lack of Love

In a remarkable study from the 1950s, 126 healthy young men were randomly selected from the Harvard graduation classes of 1952 and 1954. They were given questionnaires about their perceptions of the love they felt from their parents. Thirty-five years later, the men were followed up and 91 per cent of those who reported that they did not perceive themselves to have had warm relationships with their mothers had medically diagnosed mid-life diseases (including coronary artery disease, high blood pressure, duodenal ulcer and alcoholism). Conversely, only 45 per cent of the men who reported a warm relationship with their mothers had these health problems. Furthermore, 82 per cent of those who indicated low warmth and closeness to their fathers had these diagnoses too, compared with 50 per cent who reported high warmth and closeness. Astoundingly, 100 per cent of those who reported little warmth and closeness from either parents had diseases diagnosed in mid-life, as opposed to only 47 per cent who had warmth and closeness from both parents. In short, being loved, cared for and supported by others is critically important to our health, youthfulness and longevity.

The Importance of Self-Care

But, what if we didn't have parental love? How do we undo the damage that this may have caused? The answer to this lies once again in lifestyle medicine, so you are in the right place. All the research in the growing field of science that looks at the effects of Adverse Childhood Events (ACEs) shows that we can heal ourselves through regular self-care and self-nurturing rituals, as these send such a strong message to both our mind and body that we are deeply loved and cared for. So following the life- and health-extending practices in this book really can make a big difference!

The Value of Friendship, But Beware the "Anti-Friend"

We've already discussed briefly on page 185 how important friends are when it comes to wellbeing and leading a long, healthy life. However, this is only of value if we can tell the difference between true close friends who will be there for us through both good and bad, and friends who maybe *seem* to be fun and supportive on the surface but who make lots of little digs, make us feel uncomfortable by the way that they seem to compete with us, or leave us feeling inexplicably down after we've spent time with them. Research into the effects of these mixed-bag type of people who could be called "frenemies" ("friends" yet also "enemies") has shown that, fascinatingly, time spent with them tends to raise blood pressure more than time spent with purely negative people does. Friendships with such frenemies are known in scientific circles as "ambivalent relationships", and researchers at the University of Utah, Salt Lake City, found that having a high number of ambivalent relationships in our lives can actually be a predictor for clinically measurable depression and cardiovascular problems. So it seems that it really would be worth taking a little time out to evaluate your friendships – and figuring out whether there are any people in your life who match this description and who it would be better that you spend less time with. After all, if you want to enhance your zest and vibrancy for life, it's just as important that you work toward having fewer negative influences as well as more positive ones!

Sex

Another aspect of socialization that dramatically impacts healthy longevity is loving, connected, exciting sex. Believe it or not, whatever turns you on and works for you as part of a "good" sex life has been proven to have the capacity to actually add up to a decade of life expectancy. And the benefits of sex aren't just limited to "young people". Satisfying sex can help people in their eighties and beyond to enjoy an enhanced quality of life, too.

In fact, researchers from the Stein Institute for Research on Aging at the University of California, San Diego, found that quality of life, successful ageing and sexual satisfaction were all strongly linked – even in people aged 60 to 89+. This is particularly interesting as women traditionally seem to experience a decline in physical health (in industrialized nations) between these ages – and it is thought that maintaining a good sex life can help stave off this decline. Regular sex benefits us in a multitude of ways. It enhances cognitive function, as well as enhancing our hormone profiles. In addition, orgasms have been shown to be capable of strengthening our infection-fighting cells by approximately 20 per cent.

Sex Tips From the Ancients

The concept of sex being good for us isn't a new one. Sex is immensely important in ancient Taoist philosophy, for example, according to which deeply connected sex is believed to dramatically increase longevity. And modern research bears this out now that we know about the effects of a soup of feel-good, health-promoting neurotransmitters (including oxytocin) being produced during intimate and satisfying sex.

In Taoism, men cultivate the ability to have multiple orgasms without ejaculating so that they can preserve semen. This is because it's believed that semen production is very "costly" in terms of energy, which could lead to depletion of resources and sickness. Men can therefore be in contact for longer with their partner so that she, too, can experience multiple orgasms. You might want to look into this, as what's not to like!

The Power of the Orgasm – and Cuddling!
If a couple wants to further boost the health-enhancing benefits of sex when experiencing orgasms, it's been shown that hugging each other will do the trick, as this facilitates the excretion of the "connection hormone" oxytocin, which is directly linked to life expectancy. Believe it or not, cuddling has been shown in many studies to have the potential to increase life expectancy by as much as seven years, as well as to reduce the risk of developing depression and other chronic diseases. Don't worry if you're not with a partner, though, as no matter how you have them, orgasms are relaxing, sleep-promoting, pain-reducing and anti-inflammatory.

We are all so incredibly different. Many women never have orgasms from penetrative sex, for example, and some women report that they

Rewind Insight: Something I feel I need to share with you regarding the orgasm/age-rewind puzzle is that we women really would benefit from taking advantage of all the fun sex toys out there – and all the more so as we get older! Experimenting with dildos, vibrators and the other array of goodies available can help you to really relax and orgasm as and when it suits you. But they can also help to prevent your vaginal lining from becoming thinner and your pelvic floor muscles becoming weaker as you get older. Keeping these in shape can be an absolute game changer when it comes to not only the enjoyment of sex but also other important lifestyle issues such as urinary continence, which tends to get worse after menopause – especially if you aren't having regular sex. Many women that I have recommended sex toys to – who previously wouldn't have been at all interested (due to not knowing about their legitimate health aspects – and also because there's still so much stigma in this area!) – have told me that they now experience pain-free sex, have better muscular control and tightness, and overall, they enjoy sex so much more and therefore feel better in themselves.

simply never climax at all. If this rings true for you, rest assured that you are by no means alone.

Orgasms, as wonderful as they are, are a learned response and – given that 99 per cent of our sexual response is centered in the brain – it is crucial to get your mindset right – if, of course, having orgasms is something that feels important to you. Orgasms are complex, elusive things – and as sexual response is such a huge topic, there isn't enough space to go into everything here (we'd need another book), so I suggest that if you want to know more, you look at some of the excellent online resources about how to take full advantage of this powerfully age-reversing, deeply pleasurable and ultra-healthy human response.

So Why is Sex So Powerfully Anti-Ageing?

There are so many factors involved in sex that it is difficult for researchers to tease out what is making the most impact on our wellbeing. While we might not really know whether the "sociability factor" involved in close sexual relationships is the anti-ageing key or whether it is more to do with the sex act itself giving us a youthful boost – does it really matter?

We do know, however, that sex is a great workout – women can burn about 150 calories in a reasonably active half-hour session. (Tantric sex, which often lasts for hours on end, could be the next weight-control craze!) Aside from the huge calorie expenditure during sex, women are at another advantage in that, when we orgasm, blood floods our brains, leading to a super oxygenated state that improves our mental and emotional functions.

I strongly suspect, therefore, that it is a combination of all the various factors that make sex so good for the Rewind Your Body Clock cause: the increased blood to the brain and enhanced mental state, the host of "happy hormones" produced, the actual physical exercise, the sociability (if you're with a partner) and much more! So here's to kinder, more connected, more loving and more sensual relationships all round, as we'll all benefit as a result!

Your Relationship Mindset Moving Forward:

Now that you've come to the end of this chapter, take a little time to think about its content and come up with a specific, positive, present-tense Mindset Phrase of your own for the topic in hand, focusing on the information that has resonated most with you from the chapter.

CHAPTER 17

CONNECTING TO NATURE

> ❝ I commit to connecting to nature daily. It energizes me, and by cultivating a sense of 'awe', I am actively rewinding my body clock. ❞

We human beings are part of nature, constantly interacting with it on so many levels and in so many ways, from our tiniest molecules to our larger biological, mental, emotional and spiritual systems. Most of us know, deep down, how hugely beneficial this interaction is to us, especially with the growing prevalence of depression caused by, among other things, "nature deprivation" – due largely to the increasing amount of time we spend in front of screens, whether TVs, phones, pads or computers. We innately know that being in nature has the power to relax and refresh us. However, might there be more to it on a holistic healing and anti-ageing level?

In this chapter we will look at the positive, calming effect that being in nature has on us with a range of tips on how to deepen our connection to our natural environment. We'll also talk a little about environmental pollutants both in our home and beyond – and how to minimize the risk to ourselves and our loved ones. Lastly, we'll explore how cultivating a sense of awe at the incredible beauty of nature that surrounds us really can help us rewind our body clock and boost our health-span.

A Sense of Calm and Connection

There's already a great deal of research on the impact that nature has on our health and wellbeing; it is an exponentially growing field. This research shows that being in nature, or even viewing scenes of nature, can reduce anger, fear and stress and increase pleasant feelings and our overall sense of connection with the world around us. Being in nature also contributes to our physical health – reducing blood pressure, improving heart rate, relieving muscle tension and regulating the production of stress hormones.

Time in nature is viewed as having the power to bring us "out of ourselves" and our narrow concerns – connecting us to a wider beauty. Thus, the environment is connected not only to our physical and emotional health but also to our broader sense of meaning and purpose in life. In the results of one study published in the journal *Mind*, 95 per cent of the people interviewed reported that their mood improved after spending time outside and that they felt less stressed, anxious and depressed – and instead calmer and more balanced.

The Healing Power of Nature

Nature provides us with a welcome focus – respite from our overactive minds. And because researchers around the world have formed a consensus that we are genetically programmed to find trees, plants, water and other elements of nature completely engrossing, simply *seeing* nature scenes also has the power to distract us from pain and discomfort, and to soothe us.

This was well demonstrated in the study of patients in a suburban Pennsylvania hospital who underwent gallbladder surgery between 1972 and 1981. Half of the patients were given a view of trees from the hospital bed and the other half a view of a brick wall. Robert Ulrich, the doctor who conducted the study, found that the patients with the view of the trees tolerated pain better, had fewer negative effects from the surgery and spent less time in hospital.

More recent studies have shown similar results by only introducing *representations* of nature, such as paintings and plants, into people's surroundings. Research undertaken in hospitals, offices and schools has found that even just a simple plant in a room can cause a significant reduction in stress and anxiety levels, which in turn boosts wellbeing. What you are seeing, hearing and experiencing at any moment is changing not only your mood but how your nervous, endocrine and immune systems are responding. We understand innately that the stress of an unpleasant environment can cause us to feel anxious, sad or even helpless. Happily, a pleasing environment reverses all of that.

Nature and Sociability

As we explored in the previous chapter, one of the most profoundly important factors in remaining healthy and vibrant into our advancing years is sociability – our connection with others. Field studies conducted by Kuo and Coley over many years at the University of Illinois' Landscape and Human Health Laboratory – and published in various journals including the esteemed science journal *Nature* in 1984 – indicate that time spent in nature *also* contributes to this sense of connection as it connects us not only to each other but to the larger world, too. Another study at the University of Illinois suggests that residents in Chicago public housing who had trees and green space around the building reported knowing more people, having stronger feelings of unity with neighbours and were more concerned with helping and supporting each other. They also reported having stronger feelings of "belonging" than tenants in buildings without trees around them. In addition to this greater sense of community, they had a reduced risk of street crime, lower levels of aggression between domestic partners, and a better capacity to cope with life's demands – especially the stresses of living in poverty.

This experience of "connection" may be explained by studies that used fMRI (magnetic resonance imaging) to measure brain activity. Fascinatingly, when participants viewed nature scenes, the parts of the brain associated with empathy and love lit up, but when they viewed urban scenes, the part of the brain associated with fear and anxiety was activated, helping to explain why a lack of time spent in the natural world can sometimes be associated with a lack of empathy and altruism – and also with higher instances of depression.

How Dirt Makes Us Happy

Have you ever wondered why gardening gives so many people so much joy? Aside from the obvious rewards such as exercise, a sense of accomplishment, artistic endeavour, growing food and so on, there is another, less tangible, benefit to gardening that hasn't long been discovered. Gardening has recently been proven to make us happier due to a bacterium found in soil called *Mycobacterium vaccae*. This little bug has been found to mirror the effect on our neurons that antidepressants such as Prozac provide – but of course without the potential side effects.

The research into the connection between soil exposure, higher levels of happiness and improved relaxation was conducted on cancer patients and published in the *Annals of Oncology* in 2004. Interestingly, the patients who took part in the gardening also reported that they felt less stressed, less pain and an improved quality of life.

Researchers are now looking at whether *Mycobacterium* antidepressant microbes in soil might be able to improve cognitive function and conditions such as Crohn's disease and rheumatoid arthritis, too. The reason scientists think that these conditions could potentially be helped by exposure to this bacterium is that it causes levels of a particular cytokine (chemical messenger) to rise, which increases the production of serotonin.

So, how do we gain more exposure to *Mycobacterium vaccae* for this wellness boost? It is generally taken into our bodies through both skin contact and inhalation. This means that as dirt is dug up, or we use it to pot plants, the tiny bacteria will be dispersed into the air for us to breathe in. Plus, as we work in the soil with our hands, the physical contact allows us to further reap the benefits.

The research into this fascinating phenomenon suggests that the benefits of soil exposure can last up to three weeks – possibly more. So, if you can, get out and do some gardening in your spare time – or just get some plants and pot them up for a balcony or indoor garden. It's a fascinatingly creative way of improving all your measures of wellbeing.

The Power of Being Outdoors

As explored in Chapter 12, exercise is a key factor in enhancing wellbeing and giving you a crucial boost on your Rewind Journey. However, exercising *outdoors* has been proven to reduce stress and enhance mood significantly more than exercising indoors. In the results of a study published in the journal *Mind* in 2007, one group of participants went walking in an area where there were woods, grasslands and lakes, and another in a shopping mall. The outdoor group showed less tension, anger and depression, and better overall mood than the indoor group.

A series of fascinating studies in Japan in 2008 has also shown that walking in forests, as opposed to urban environments, lowered blood pressure and stress hormones well beyond the time of the walk.

So, any time you have the chance, make a little time to go somewhere with trees, grass, flowers, water or other natural elements and enjoy a walk, run or cycle in order to give yourself a wellness boost. And if you live in an urban environment, just go to your local park or green space.

Even if you can only get out for five or ten minutes during your lunch hour to get a breath of fresh air and give your mind a break, you will reap the rewards of feeling more grounded and having more energy afterwards.

And if you can't get out into nature as much as you would like, then a good alternative is to bring some aspects of nature inside instead, so see below for a range of ideas on this.

REWIND PRACTICE – OVER TO YOU
Bring Nature Into Your Home

- Open the curtains as much as possible: Letting in natural light enhances productivity, boosts satisfaction levels and reduces depression. It can also help to enhance recovery from illness and accidents. An interesting study compared the use of pain medications in patients who were on the bright versus the dim side of a hospital. Those on the bright side reported less stress and pain, and needed fewer analgesics.
- Introduce plants to your living space: Adding a few plants to your home can boost wellbeing on many levels, including reducing the amount of airborne pollutants. Research done in the 1970s and '80s by NASA demonstrated the air-cleansing powers of plants in the Skylab biospheres.
- Embrace aromatherapy: Nature is full of wonderful plant aromas, which can be used in the form of essential oils not only to make our surroundings smell delightful, but also to enhance our thinking, mood, immune system and more. Increasing numbers of scientists are looking at the therapeutic effect of different plant oils on various health conditions. Two examples supported by research looked at peppermint oil, which has been shown to enhance attention and lessen mental and physical fatigue, and lavender oil, which has been proven to have calming qualities. Try using a few drops of either of these in an oil diffuser at home to enhance your mood.
- Add visual depictions of nature scenes: If you don't have a view of nature from a window at home or work, you can still benefit from its rejuvenating powers by adding a painting or photo of the natural world to your space. Find one that you really like. Some researchers hypothesize that we might instinctively prefer a view of an open landscape rather than a forest, as, in more primitive times, an open landscape would have been less stressful in terms of being able to see any predators lurking. This is thought to be a throwback to our hunter-gatherer ancestry.

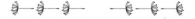

Rewind Insight: A large body of research shows that there are great all-round wellness benefits to spending time with animals or owning a pet, including the potential for lower blood pressure and less anxiety and depression. Plus, if the animal happens to be one that needs to be walked, you have a built-in exercise programme too, and the perfect excuse to get out and about outdoors!

Environmental Toxicity

While we're talking about the impact of nature in our lives, it's really worthwhile to take stock of the many toxins in our environment these days that can cause premature ageing and potential health problems, from hormonal disruption (discussed in Chapter 15) to breathing difficulties.

I've noticed in my complementary health practice that a lot of people have been coming to me in recent years with all sorts of "strange" conditions that nobody can really seem to explain in conventional medical terms, including allergies, headaches, depression, unexplained weight gain and much more – conditions that didn't seem as prevalent in the past.

Practitioners in a branch of healthcare called Environmental Medicine believe that it's the modern environmental stressors that we are exposed to on a continual basis that are the underlying factor in the huge growth of these conditions. Although there is, of course, a huge *variety* of stressors and polluters, we are going to take a look at two of the most prominent of these – namely environmental pollution, caused by petrochemicals and other chemical contaminants, and electro smog, caused by Wi-Fi, TVs, cell phones, computers and other devices that give off radiation.

Environmental Pollution

External environmental pollution caused by factors such as smog presents a serious health problem; the World Health Organization has data showing that things like this shorten our lifespan. This makes it really crucial for us to take any actions we can to lessen any such pollution.

However, a more insidious problem exists within our homes, where we are constantly surrounded by artificially produced items that exude chemicals. These items include furniture, carpeting, paint, upholstery and even our food, which often contains all sorts of pesticides. The colourless and odourless poisons that are on, in and exuded by these items have become a "normal" part of our lives over the past 30–40 years; our exposure to them is relentless. And while acute exposure to chemical substances can cause an immediate reaction, such as allergies, which, while inconvenient and uncomfortable, very often will not do any long-lasting damage to our overall health, unfortunately, continued exposure over a longer period of time can be much more dangerous as symptoms accumulate in the background, potentially "unseen" for decades. Exposure to such chemicals can, over time, compromise our immune system in particular, which, in turn, makes it much more of a struggle to remain healthy in the first place. And there is now strong evidence to suggest that chronic exposure to synthetic chemicals is actually likely to shorten our lifespans, which means it is wise to reduce the use of these chemicals as much as possible (see below).

REWIND PRACTICE – OVER TO YOU
Improve Your Home Environment

Below are a range of suggested ways in which you can start to reduce the amount of synthetic chemicals in your everyday environment and therefore make your relationship with your surroundings a healthier one:

- Inform yourself about traditional, natural cleaning products, such as white vinegar, lemon juice and baking soda. As well as being non-toxic, these are good value and really work! (Beware of shop-bought cleaning agents that claim to contain "natural" ingredients, as these claims don't always stand up to scrutiny.)
- Use non-biological washing powder or, even better, look into natural alternatives such as washing balls (a large plastic ball with small stone balls, ceramic beads and other objects inside – designed to agitate your washing better, thus getting it clean without the need for chemicals).
- Choose organic decorating materials when you next update your home as standard paints are loaded with potential hormone disruptors.
- Source furniture and furnishings made from natural materials when you're next buying new items for your home.

Electro Smog

"Electro smog" is the collective term used for the electromagnetic fields (EMFs) that are created by emissions from man-made sources, such as radio wave signals, microwaves, Wi-Fi and mobile phone masts. Although their negative effects have not yet been *definitively* proven, these frequencies are believed by an increasing number of both scientists and lay people to be potentially extremely harmful.

EMFs have a resonance that is completely out of sync with our body's *natural* resonance, yet we're not all affected by EMFs to the same degree, with some of us being much more sensitive to them. However, whichever end of this spectrum you're on, it really is wise to reduce your exposure to sources such as mobile phones, transmitters and electricity supply lines, all of which could potentially contribute toward health problems in the long term. I personally believe that we won't fully understand the damage that devices likes these cause until several decades into the future, but in the meantime it would make good sense to protect ourselves against any future damage now, so below are some ideas for doing this.

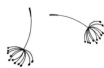

REWIND PRACTICE – OVER TO YOU
Reduce Your EMF Device Usage

It will take a little time and effort to cleanse your environment of toxins, so start small. In the short term, de-clutter your environment, getting rid of anything that you suspect might cause you problems.

A few top tips are to unplug as many items as you can, turn off your Wi-Fi at night, and never sleep with your mobile phone switched on and near you.

It's important, however, not to get in any way stressed out by the thought of toxin exposure. Just address the issue step by step, as stress would only be a *hindrance* to the long, healthy, happy, vibrant life you're in search of. So, if ever you find yourself feeling overwhelmed by it, just throw open your windows, let the sunshine in, treat yourself to a beautiful bunch of flowers, put your favourite music on and simply delight in nature and in life, knowing that you're doing the very best you can.

The Power of Being Awe-Struck

A lot of research has been done in recent years on the effect of positive emotions such as awe on our holistic health and wellbeing. People's responses to beauty in both nature and the arts have been given particular focus, such as views of the Grand Canyon, walking through a beautiful forest, listening to Schubert's "Ave Maria" or viewing great works of art like the Sistine Chapel. Such awesome stimuli were shown to provoke positive emotional responses in the people being studied that led to them producing lower levels of pro-inflammatory cytokines – the hormonal messengers that "tell" our bodies to ramp up our inflammatory response so that our immune system will work harder when it views itself as being under threat. As the lead researcher on this study, Dr Jennifer Stellar explained, "Our findings demonstrate that positive emotions are associated with the markers of good health."

Cytokines are necessary for launching this protective immune response, swiftly directing cells to our body's battlegrounds in order to fight disease. Under normal circumstances this is helpful and can even be life-saving. However, it has only recently been discovered that elevated levels of pro-inflammatory cytokines can have a negative effect on us emotionally. In fact, elevated pro-inflammatory cytokines has been tied to depression. Many studies have now found that patients suffering from depression had higher levels of the cytokine known as TNF-alpha than their non-depressed counterparts. It is currently believed that by signalling the brain to produce inflammatory molecules, these cytokines can block key hormones and neurotransmitters – such as serotonin and dopamine – t hat control moods, appetite, sleep and memory.

How "Awe" Can Combat Chronic Inflammation

The fact that the sense of awe we feel when viewing scenes of great beauty has been shown to promote healthier levels of cytokines suggests that anything we can do to experience this emotion – whether a walk in nature, watching the sun set or losing ourselves in a piece of music – has the capacity to influence our health and our life expectancy.

Two separate experiments were conducted in which over 200 young adults reported on a given day the extent to which they had experienced positive emotions such as compassion, contentment, joy, love, pride, awe, wonder and amazement. Swab samples of inner cheek tissue that had been taken that same day showed that those who experienced more of these positive emotions, especially awe, wonder and amazement, had the lowest levels of the cytokine "Interleukin 6" (IL6), which is a marker of inflammation.

So, why should awe be such a predictor of reduced pro-inflammatory cytokines? The latest studies suggest that this emotion seems to be related to curiosity and a desire within us to explore our environment. As for which came first – the low pro-inflammatory cytokines or the positive feelings – scientists don't know for sure: it's possible that having lower inflammatory cytokines makes us experience more positive emotions, or, conversely, that positivity reduces these particular cytokine levels.

Either way, what we do know is that it would be fantastic for all of us to get out into nature more and take the time to truly and deeply nurture both ourselves and the natural environment around us, to keep us in the best shape possible.

Your Nature Mindset Moving Forward:

Now that you've come to the end of this chapter, take a little time to think about its content and come up with a specific, positive, present-tense Mindset Phrase of your own for the topic in hand, focusing on the information that has resonated most with you from the chapter.

CHAPTER 18
RESTFUL SLEEP

> ❝ I know that good sleep has vast benefits that support my health in all respects. I actively cultivate excellent sleep habits, ensuring that I get the right amount of sleep for me. ❞

Confession time: I'm writing this chapter as a reformed insomniac. I have struggled with sleep my entire life. My dad did too, and yet my mum can quite happily sleep on a fence. (So unfair!)

Living with chronic insomnia is brutal, as it affects every area of your life, and it is my deepest wish that this chapter will help you if you are suffering – or enable you to share the information with friends and loved ones if they are. Equally, even if your sleep patterns are decent but you feel they could be enhanced to help you feel more generally rested, I hope you will find something in this chapter for you, too.

The difference it makes to your life when you get sleep under control and feel more rejuvenated is profound. In fact, I wish sleep skills were taught in schools as there's no doubt that good "sleep hygiene" – by which I mean achieving factors such as the length, depth and quality of sleep that is right for you, as an individual – is one of the most important life skills there is, and dramatically impacts how you both look, feel and function.

In this chapter, we'll look at the many benefits of good sleep and how it's connected to rewinding your biological body clock. We'll also discuss the importance of respecting the body's natural rhythms and some of the problems associated with poor sleep patterns, and, finally, I'll share a range of tips and techniques with you to help you get more consistent, deeply restful and restorative sleep, so that you can both look and feel your best, whatever your age.

Beauty Sleep

So, is the notion of "needing your beauty sleep" a real thing? Does lack of sleep really affect how we look? I'm afraid to say the answer to both those questions is a resounding "yes"! Getting enough consistent sleep is vital when it comes to looking and feeling better: it gives us both an outer and an inner glow. But it goes much deeper than that. Sleep isn't just a passive thing that happens to us, during which we are inert; rather, it is a very active time, metabolically speaking, with much more going on than we often realize, as you'll learn throughout this chapter.

The Health Benefits of Sleep

Getting good rest enables our brain to work faster and better, enhances the performance of our heart and circulatory systems, and so much more. It's even been shown to improve telomere length, which, as we know from Chapter 2 (page 42), has the capacity to make us "biologically" younger!

Aside from the general physical and metabolic renewal and repair that goes on, research suggests that our brain actually cleanses itself during deeper phases of sleep, sorting through the emotions we've experienced during the day just past, and it's hypothesized that "arranging" things in this way may facilitate recall and learning.

It is also during deep sleep that our HGH (Human Growth Hormone) production is at its highest. And, as we know from Chapter 12, HGH plays a crucial role in healthy ageing and improved metabolism. In fact, it has been shown that good sleep in young adulthood through to middle age can help to protect us from cognitive decline in later years.

The benefits of consistently getting a "good night's sleep" are too numerous to go into detail on *all* of them. I've therefore chosen a few of the *key* ones for exploration in the pages that follow, as, in my opinion, these are among the factors most relevant to feeling and functioning as vitally and vibrantly as possible on your Rewind Journey.

Healthy Weight Control

When it comes to maintaining a healthy weight – and particularly staving off the development of toxic visceral fat, which, as we know, is associated with the dramatic increase of pro-inflammatory chemicals and potential premature ageing – getting a consistently good amount of sleep is vital.

Poor sleep is deeply detrimental to the way that our metabolism functions. It also increases hunger as we produce a hormone called ghrelin when we are sleep-deprived. This pushes our hunger and need for calorie intake into overdrive. Historically, ghrelin was vital to our survival because it drove our ancestors to find food – and it helped them to maintain a healthy level of body fat. However, these days, we could do without it gnawing away at us, telling us to eat more. In fact, ghastly ghrelin tricks our metabolism into behaving as if we are in starvation mode when we're sleep-deprived – so, in an elevated ghrelin state, the foods with the highest fat and sugar content suddenly become the most attractive to us! It's at this point when all we want to do is to bring on the doughnuts; fresh juices and kale just won't cut it! When we're well rested, on the other hand, it becomes so much easier to make good food choices and therefore keep our weight-related health in check.

Heart Health

Heart disease still remains the leading cause of mortality in both men and women in industrialized nations, although deaths from cancer are fast catching up. And good sleep habits are associated with reducing the underlying causes of cardiovascular disease. Even short-term sleep deprivation has been shown to elevate blood pressure and to predispose us to frightening events such as having a heart attack or a stroke.

In a study of nearly 72,000 female nurses (see NursesHealthStudy.org for a full overview of this fascinating data), researchers found that both sleeping too little and too much was correlated with higher risks of developing heart disease over a ten-year period as compared with normal sleepers. And the risk of cardiovascular problems associated with sleep deprivation don't just affect the middle-aged and elderly; even teenagers who have poor sleep exhibit evidence of metabolic change and a predisposition to cardiovascular disease.

Ability to Deal With Stress

Have you ever had the experience of facing a challenge, not really knowing quite what to do about it and someone telling you to "sleep on it"? Well, it turns out that this is wise advice – because what we are seeing in research now is that adequate sleep really does influence our ability to process thoughts and emotions, as well as refining our ability to react to stimuli in an appropriate manner.

This means that, when well rested, we have the capacity to react in much more measured ways to stressful situations, we are likely to feel less overwhelmed, we are more likely to display patience, we will be capable of far better decision-making and we are less likely to fly off the handle at relatively unimportant matters!

Enhanced Memory

Sleep affects our memory in various ways, not least how we process and archive new memories, how we access old memories and how accurate our recall ability is. It has been shown that when we are lacking in sleep, we are much more susceptible to false memories and more likely to remember things that happened to us in the past as being more negative than we perceived them at the time.

Altered Behaviour

There's also evidence to suggest that we are more prone to increased anger and aggression when sleep-deprived. And yet more research shows that our relationships with our friends, family and partners may suffer when we're exhausted as we are less able to interpret one another's emotions correctly.

Perhaps most worryingly, lack of sleep has also been shown to have the potential to actually start to alter our moral judgement. In a research study on nurses, published in the scientific journal *Sleep* in 2007, it was found that those who were sleep-deprived were more likely to be rude or aggressive to others, or even to lie and steal. They were also less conscientious with caring tasks and medication administration.

Taking all of this into consideration, it becomes all the more obvious that sleep really is a topic to be taken seriously if you want to stay happy, healthy and in loving relationships with those around you for as long as possible. So let's now look at what we mean by a "good" amount of sleep and rest.

How Much Sleep?

There have been some notable characters in history who have been able to not just survive but seemingly *thrive* on very little sleep, such as British Prime Minister Winston Churchill during the World War Two years, but it is estimated that such people comprise only about 3 per cent of the population. For most people, all the research suggests that seven to eight hours' sleep a night is a healthy average in order to function optimally.

Having said this, the fact that we are, of course, all unique means that different people will have differing needs depending on a wide range of factors from age and life circumstances to current stress levels. If you are under stress, for example – whether physical, mental or emotional – you may find that you need more sleep, or rest of another form.

Rise and Shine

In order to begin my day as healthily as possible, I like to use a "healthy waking" alarm app on my cell phone that works by monitoring my breathing patterns throughout the night, so that it can work out a time to waken me when I am optimally refreshed. So, for example, if you need to be up by, say, 6.30 a.m., it will remind you when to go to bed based on how many hours of sleep you tell it you would like. It will then monitor your body to detect when you are at the lightest point in your sleep cycle and waken you within a half-hour slot before your desired wake time. This way, you are much less likely to feel groggy than if an alarm suddenly sounds out of the blue when you are maybe in your deepest phase of sleep. It's very clever and, for me, it really does work!

There is now quite a range of science-based apps like this that offer health-enhancing sleep services, so why not do a little research into them and see if any of them might suit you? Please note, though, that I strongly recommend that you put your phone onto "aeroplane" mode if you do choose to use a phone-based sleep app; we discussed the dangers of EMFs in Chapter 17. Otherwise, if you prefer a non-digital approach, or if you would simply prefer not to keep your phone by your bed at night (which is definitely good "sleep hygiene" practice), other ways to be wakened in a less harsh way than an annoying ring tone, loud buzzer or piercing bleep of some sort include alarms with radio, music or birdsong options and also alarms with lights that come on gradually over a chosen time period, mimicking the gentle, rejuvenating effect of a sunrise.

Tuning Into Our Own Needs

Dr Ernest Rossi, the respected US psychologist, discovered through his extensive research that, on the whole, we humans are able to be fairly well focused for up to 90 minutes before we tail off into a 20-minute lull. This lull is believed by Rossi and his colleagues to be a healing break – where your brain processes information that has gone before and cleanses itself.

In his outstanding book called *The 20-Minute Break*, Rossi explains how to recognize and reorganize your natural rhythms to optimize your performance – and your health – throughout the day. His idea, in line with the findings mentioned above, is that every 90 minutes or so, you should take a 20-minute break to avoid getting tired and irritable, losing your mental focus, making mistakes and maybe even having accidents – and, ultimately, to avoid becoming stressed to the point that you get sick. He explains that by doing this you are respecting an internal body clock function known as ultradian rhythms – natural cycles that *recur* throughout a 24-hour period – thus helping yourself avoid a condition known as the Ultradian Stress Syndrome, which is akin to "burnout".

Taking Regular Breaks

I have worked out that the best pattern for me personally is as follows: After my morning start-up routine of yoga stretches, meditation, shower etc., I start work at about 9 a.m. and work until 10.30 a.m. I then have a 20-minute break for a cup of tea and maybe a snack. This is my "ultradian" break, so it's important that I put my phone down, get away from my computer and don't do anything taxing to my mind during this time.

I then get back to work, feeling refreshed and re-energized, and after another 90 minutes, I take another 20-minute break. Again, I don't do anything mentally demanding during this time – perhaps go for a walk, grab something to eat, put on a meditation recording or listen to hypnosis track. I find that if I organize my entire day like this, I am able to focus much more intently, and I get a lot more done.

Why not try to monitor your own performance and rhythms throughout each day to see if you can work out when it best works for you to take restorative breaks? They will make a huge difference to your wellbeing as well as your productivity! It can even be useful to keep a diary to track how different patterns make you feel in order to assess what really works best for you.

Circadian Rhythms

We really shouldn't be talking about sleep without mentioning the all-important circadian rhythms – our 24-hour internal cycles that are so important that the 2017 Nobel Prize in Physiology or Medicine was awarded to a team of researchers who elicited the molecular mechanisms that control them. The word "circadian" comes from the Latin *circum*, which means "around", and *dies*, which means "day". This "body clock" – seated deep within every cell of our body (including our brain) – has hard-wired the rotation of the earth into the very fabric of our cells over countless millennia.

We are all aware of the temporal ebb and flow of the rhythms that shape our days. The most basic of these that we live by is the sleep–wake cycle, which is related to the cycle of the sun when in balance:

- As our internal clock senses evening hours coming on, a signal is sent to increase melatonin levels and encourage sleep.
- Then, just before dawn, another array of hormonal messengers begin to surge, readying us for wakefulness and the beginning of the day.

The Importance of Darkness

When melatonin is secreted in response to our environment getting darker, it helps to make us feel sleepy. It's for this reason that it's advised to sleep in darkness when possible – because, if light intrudes, melatonin production stops, disrupting our sleep cycle.

It's also advised not to use screens just before bed – or while in bed – if you want consistently good sleep as the blue light that they emit disrupts the darkness, suppressing our melatonin production and causing all sorts of potential issues, including insomnia.

Conversely, if you have difficulty waking, you can buy special blue-light emitting devices that suppress melatonin in the *morning* and help you to wake and be more energetic; these devices can also be helpful for anyone who suffers from Seasonal Affective Disorder.

Sleep Scheduling

When it comes to the specific times during which you sleep, there's no magical one-size-fits-all schedule. The best approach is simply to choose your sleep times to match your own physiological rhythms in order to get the recommended seven to eight hours. With a bit of experimenting, you should be able to work out what is best for you.

Rewind Insight: Some natural nutritional sources of melatonin for you to take in the evening if you would like to encourage your body into relaxation mode include the following (it's best to take them about half an hour before you wish to sleep):

- Bananas
- Tart cherries
- Dark leafy greens
- Hummus
- Nuts

The Effect of Disrupted Sleep Patterns

Factors such as jetlag, overwork, extreme stress and shift work tend to throw our normal sleep patterns out, and even shifting the clock an hour forward or backward to adjust for daylight saving time can considerably disrupt our biological clock. For example, it's been shown that workplace injuries and traffic accidents are more frequent when we lose an hour of sleep after a clock change, and in a study published in the *British Medical Journal's Open Heart* in 2014, heart patients were shown to be at greater risk of myocardial infarction the week after the daylight saving time shift.

Sleep and Circadian Rhythm Disruption

A condition known as "Sleep and Circadian Rhythm Disruption" (SCRD) can occur when our natural circadian rhythms are pushed out of sync to an extreme degree. This is a feature shared by some of the most challenging diseases of our time – from serious eye disorders and Alzheimer's to bipolar disorder and schizophrenia. Its symptoms can include difficulty getting to sleep, difficulty staying asleep, non-restorative sleep, impaired performance during waking hours (including a decrease in cognitive skills), daytime sleepiness and poor concentration.

Compounds that encourage the inflammatory response connected to SCRD rise at night, explaining why we often feel worse in the evening if we are ill, and those that inhibit it rise during the day. This is likely to be because our body is better at combatting infection while at rest and, thus, energy can be recruited for healing, rather than being channelled into other functions. Furthermore, activity of our stress-response system – particularly the secretion of the stress hormone, cortisol – is reduced during night-time hours and heightened in the early morning. This is one of the reasons why people with the painful condition rheumatoid arthritis feel so much worse in the morning: excessively elevated cortisol – and thus increased inflammation – causes their joints to be more painful and stiff.

Thankfully, scientists are making huge advances in ascertaining more about how our body's constellation of internal timekeepers interact with, and help govern, the function of our bodily systems and how this impacts our overall vitality. And it's clear from this that keeping your body's daily sleep cycle balanced may be one of the best things you can do for your health. In the pages that follow I therefore share some tried-and-tested suggestions with you – including Ayurvedic teachings on sleep and a yogic approach to establishing healthy sleep called "Yoga Nidra".

Sleep Tips From Ancient Ayurveda

Ayurvedic medicine is a holistic ancient Indian approach to wellbeing that has healthy longevity as one of its core tenets. Here follows a range of simple, positive habits encouraged in Ayurvedic philosophy to enhance good sleep which I have adopted myself and which have totally transformed my sleep – and life! Goodbye insomnia – and good riddance!

• Get enough sleep: Eight hours are recommended in Ayurveda, which is similar to what is recommended by modern Western researchers. But it is believed that people who are ill, pregnant or elderly may need more.

• Develop a regular sleep schedule: In Ayurveda, it is believed that it is ideal to go to bed early (ideally 90 minutes after sunset) and to wake up early, too (ideally, 90 minutes before sunset). This can be tricky if you are living in the far northern or southern hemispheres, as, in the summer months, you'd get far too little sleep. However, regularity of bedtime, sleep duration and waking time is key, so try to set your alarm to wake you at the same time every day. After a while, your body's rhythms will begin to fit in with the schedule you've set, and you'll find that you'll automatically want to go to bed at the same time each night.

• Work with your Ayurvedic mind–body type called your *dosha*. This is your own unique blend of physical, emotional and mental characteristics. The three primary *doshas* are listed below, each with a different sleep pattern recommended for it. See if you recognize yourself in any of these, bearing in mind that it is possible to be a *combination*.
    Vata (air or wind types): Vata people tend to be the typical ectomorph, with long, lean limbs and prominent joints. They tend to have dry skin and can suffer from dry eyes and sometimes be constipated. They are energetic, active, bright, talkative and emotional. Vata people dream a lot as they process a lot of their emotional experiences during the sleep state. They therefore tend to need 8–10 hours' sleep. It can help Vata people to sleep more comfortably if they have a softer bed as they can be quite bony.
    Pitta (fire types): Pitta people tend to be mesomorphs – quite well-built, who can gain muscle and strength easily. They may tend toward oily skin, they are flexible and they often have sensitivities and allergies. Personality-wise, they are strong, organized leaders. They need a moderate amount of 7–8 hours' sleep and tend to do well on a medium mattress (neither too soft, nor too hard).

213

Kapha (water types): Kapha types tend to be endomorphs, with a substantial build, who can gain weight easily. Kapha people are methodical and even-tempered, and show great patience. Family and friends are hugely important to them. Because they tend to find it easy to sleep, they don't need quite as much as the other categories: 7 hours or sometimes a little less. They do well on a firm mattress.

- Don't eat just before sleep: Ayurvedic practitioners recommend not eating anything for at least an hour or two before bed as the digestive process interferes with the body's ability to rest fully. Going for a gentle evening walk after your dinner can also be really helpful as it regulates blood sugar, which is considered beneficial for sleep promotion.

- Choose your sleeping position well: In Ayurvedic tradition, we are advised to "Sleep on the left side, wake up on the right". Falling asleep on our left side is believed to position the stomach ideally for good sleep and also to facilitate liver function as it doesn't press down on your liver (which sits on the right side of your body). It also leaves your right nostril more open to breathe through, which, in Ayurveda, is connected to the idea of completing things and is therefore viewed as more restful. When you wake up in the morning, turn over to your right side and rest there for a few minutes before getting up. This now encourages you to breathe through your left nostril, associated with thinking and creating, in order to wake up your brain, as well as stimulating the peristaltic motion of your bowels from the transverse colon to the descending colon, which will create an urge to go to the bathroom.

- Massage your feet before sleep: In Ayurveda, massaging your feet is believed to "ground" you, making you feel more relaxed and at ease, and therefore more ready for sleep. Personally, I like to use coconut oil for this and think about just how much my feet have done for me that day – as a token of love and appreciation for carrying me around.

- Make a soothing bedtime drink: I like to follow this traditional Ayurvedic recipe as it really helps send me off to the Land of Nod: Mix about 240ml (9fl oz) water, 60g (2oz /½ cup) cashews, 60g (2oz) turmeric root, a little saffron and a hint of black pepper in a high-speed blender until it warms up. If you don't have a high-speed blender, just mix in a normal blender until smooth, then warm up in a saucepan.

- Try the "One-Minute Sleep Challenge" below – a yoga breathing technique that is said, with regular practice, to have the power to help you fall asleep in less than a minute once you go to bed!

REWIND PRACTICE – OVER TO YOU
One-Minute Sleep Challenge

Often known as the 4, 7, 8 technique, this deeply relaxing breathing technique, with its roots in ancient Indian tradition, was popularized in the West by Dr Andrew Weil. It has recently been doing the rounds on the internet as a "challenge" – a bit like the "ice-bucket challenge" but nicer, you'll learn, as the potential result is beautifully restful sleep.

Note: The tongue position in the first step can feel a bit awkward to begin with, and all the more so when you breathe out through your mouth in Step 4 with your tongue still in place. But you'll know that you're doing it correctly if your breath makes a sound like a "whoosh" as the air escapes.

1. Sit up straight and rest the tip of your tongue on your gum line, just behind your upper front teeth. Keep it here throughout the process.
2. With your mouth closed, breathe in gently through your nose for a count of four.
3. Retain your breath for a count of seven. This breath hold is thought to oxygenate the blood and help the nervous system transition into a more predominantly parasympathetic mode.
4. Breathe out fully through your mouth for a count of eight, with your tongue still in place on your upper gum line. There should be a whooshing sound as the air escapes.
5. Repeat for a total of four rounds.

People who have been taking the challenge say that you get the best results if you do the exercise twice a day, morning and evening, for a couple of months. I would attest to that as it has worked for me too! I couldn't quite say that it makes me fall asleep in one minute every night, but I certainly don't struggle as much with getting off to sleep as I used to!

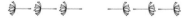

REWIND PRACTICE – OVER TO YOU

Relax with Yoga Nidra

I'd like to end this section of the book by sharing with you a deeply powerful relaxation exercise called Yoga Nidra. This is one of the most profoundly healing, and therefore anti-ageing, activities that I know and is my "go-to" technique for falling asleep fast – and staying asleep.

It is said to give you the equivalent of two hours' restorative sleep in just a 20-minute session – a tall claim but one I'm happy to agree with, as it certainly tends to feel that way when you do it!

It can be done any time of the day or night that you feel frazzled and in need of some relaxation, but it is particularly useful if you're struggling to get to sleep. I use it virtually every night before I go to bed.

Yoga Nidra is a deep, experiential process, so it works best if you don't over-think the steps. You are likely to get the best result by listening to a recording, such as the one that I have made available to download from my website, JayneyGoddard.org. Clients of mine who have used this often joke that they've no idea how it ends – or even if it has an ending! – as it is so deeply relaxing that they drift right off. I'm more than happy with that feedback. In fact, I consider that "job done"! However, if you would rather try the technique now, here follows some step-by-step guidance:

1. Lie down in a comfortable position, ensuring you won't be disturbed for 20 minutes. Turn off your phone and acknowledge to yourself that this is time for you to recharge your energy and to deeply rest your body. This is a sacred rite that honours your total wellbeing. Make sure you are warm, and move around a little to get as comfortable as possible. Sink deeper into the ground and settle in. Remind yourself that this is time for you. Everything is OK. There's nothing to do other than this rite – for yourself. There's nowhere to go and nothing that needs your attention right now. All you are doing is lying down, relaxing and listening. All is calm.

2. Come into stillness now and gently rest, allowing your body to sink into the ground or whatever surface you are lying upon, and feeling your bones becoming heavy. Release them further and deeper.

3. Set your intention for this time of deep relaxation. What is your heart's deepest desire? What is your innermost longing? Phrase it positively in the present tense. Everyone's desires are different, so just choose

your own – there is no right or wrong. It might be something like "I am relaxed and peaceful; my body is healing in every way." Once you have created your own personal and meaningful intention, repeat it three times as though it has already manifested into the present moment.

4. Starting at the top of your head and working down through your body, we will now begin a body scan. You are simply going to travel through your body at a medium pace, with awareness – acknowledging each part, in turn, with love and gratitude, welcoming all sensation, accepting everything that arises without judgement, allowing yourself time to sense each part of your body but moving on to the next part without lingering for *too* long. So start by observing the crown of your head, then gradually move to your forehead, the right side of your head, the back of your head, the left side of your head, your right temple, your left temple, your right eye, your left eye, your eye sockets, your nose – right nostril, left nostril. Next, your mouth – how does your mouth feel? Sense your upper lip, lower lip, chin and jaw. What is the feeling where your lips meet? Sense the roof of your mouth, gums, upper and lower teeth, tongue (both at the centre and at the root), inner cheeks and outer cheeks. Feel all the parts together as a whole. Feel your entire head and face as pure, vibrant, radiating, shimmering energy. Work through your whole body in this way – gently, calmly – sensing and acknowledging each part internally and externally, just observing sensation, and allowing it simply to be.

5. Restate your heartfelt intention from Step 3 three times as though it has already manifested into the present moment. Then become aware of your breath, allowing it to come and go naturally, effortlessly. As it flows through you, observe its movement. Note the ebb and flow, like gentle waves breaking on the shore – no effort needed, simply allowing it to happen. As you inhale, observe the way that a clear, fresh wave of energy and light flows upward throughout your entire body, cleansing, calming and healing every single cell. Let your cells shimmer and sparkle with the clear, clean, healthy energy that comes with each breath. Each exhalation allows anything no longer needed to float away, drifting away so that your entire body, mind and being is calm, clear, healing and serene.

6. **(a) If you wish to carry on with your day**
    When you feel ready, allow yourself to begin to return to a more normal, everyday sense of awareness, gently wriggling your fingers and

toes, perhaps having a good stretch. Cover your eyes with your hands and then open your eyes, allowing the light to filter in through your fingers. Eventually, when you are ready, roll onto your right side – into a foetal position. Rest there a little longer and, finally, and only when you are ready, gently ease yourself up into a seated position. Remember that the Yoga Nidra session that you have just experienced goes very deep and is profoundly healing, so take your time before rising to your feet as sometimes people can feel dizzy if they get up too quickly.

OR b) If you want to go to sleep

If you are still awake after Step 6, simply acknowledge to yourself that you would like to sleep now – giving yourself permission to gently drift off when you are ready.

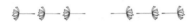

Your Restful Sleep Mindset Moving Forward:

Now that you've come to the end of this chapter, take a little time to think about its content and come up with a specific, positive, present-tense Mindset Phrase of your own for the topic in hand, focusing on the information that has resonated most with you from the chapter.

PART III

YOUR 21-DAY REWIND PLAN

Taking Immediate Action

"Knowing is not enough, you must apply; willing is not enough, you must do."
Bruce Lee

In this, the final section of this book, I would like to share with you a 21-day plan that I hope you will find useful as a means of getting you well and truly into a vibrant Rewind mindset and therefore actively kickstarting your Rewind Journey.

You will see that, after encouraging you to take a little time to reassess your motivations and goals, and being sure that you have a range of positive habits in place to build into each day and week as a base practice, the 21-day plan itself is split into three weeks, each with its own distinct theme:

• Week 1: Simplifying, Detoxing and Decluttering
• Week 2: Building, Growing and Expanding
• Week 3: Consolidating, Strengthening and Sustaining

To me, these themes are the key stages in any journey of growth and transformation, which is what, of course, I hope this plan takes you on in your quest to rewind your body clock – and feel younger in not just body but mind and spirit, too.

You can start the plan on any day of the week, at any time of the year, so I urge you not to put it off. Why not start today and begin to live life as you mean to continue – more consciously, more vibrantly and, ultimately, more in control of your own health, happiness and longevity?

It is my most sincere wish that you benefit as much from applying both this 21-day plan and all the tips and exercises from throughout the book in *your* life as I have from applying them to mine!

GETTING STARTED

WELCOME TO YOUR
21-DAY PLAN!

When you have a plan to work to, everything in life seems simpler and a lot more achievable – because you have a blueprint for success! In the pages that follow is the 21-day, or 3-week, blueprint that I have created as a starting point for you to launch yourself on your Rewind Journey.

In each of the weekly sections – which are based on the themes of simplifying, detoxing and decluttering; building, growing and expanding; consolidating, strengthening and sustaining – you will find:

- Firstly a little insight into the underlying sense of the theme and how it can help you achieve your goals.
- Next, some advice on nutrition and supplements to support you on this stage of your journey.
- Last but not least, a suggested list of varied activities for each of the seven days of that week, some of which are taken directly from the content you've already read and many of which are new but which complement and underpin all the suggestions and activities from throughout the book; these can be done in any order desired.

Please bear in mind that, while this plan has been designed as a springboard toward your Rewind goals, the lists of suggestions are in no way meant to be prescriptive. Ultimately, the ideas are for you to choose from as feels best for you – and for you to add to from the rest of the book in line with your own health and longevity requirements, which I hope you've become more familiar with as you've worked through the chapters of the book.

Even if you haven't yet read the rest of the book, please do feel free to give the 21-day plan a go if it appeals to you; it might just be the push you need to then take things further and explore some of the other tips in the book and beyond. And if you *have* read the rest of the book, then thank you and well done!

Knowing Your Motivation

Before diving into the day-by-day practical plan, let's take a look back at the lists you created as part of the "Setting Your Motivations and Goals" Rewind Practice on page 17. Do you still feel in alignment with what you wrote then? If so, great. But if any of your priorities have changed, it's no problem – just alter them as required. Knowing exactly what is motivating you will be seriously helpful in keeping you on track with the plan and in preventing distractions from steering you off course.

Knowing Your Own Mind

Now turn your attention to the Mindset Phrases that you were asked to create at the end of each chapter in Part II of the book, as per the guidance on page 16. If you haven't already done so, it is very useful to write these down all in one place, whether in a notebook, your journal, or even in the dedicated space that I have provided on my website, JayneyGoddard.org. Or, if you'd rather work with the Mindset Phrases that I provided for you at the *start* of each chapter in Part II, then write these ones down instead.

Then just take a few moments to read through this list and circle the ones that feel the most important to you, and/or that you feel you need to pay the most attention to in order to be successful in your quest to look, feel and *be* more vibrant and youthful. You could even write out your favourite ones on stickie notes and pin or place them somewhere around your home so that you will regularly see them – perhaps on the refrigerator door, on your computer, on the bathroom mirror, or in your bag – to help keep you in a positive, "can-do" frame of mind about whichever aspects of health and longevity you choose to focus on right now.

Adopting Positive Habits

When you're starting off on any new journey, it can be incredibly helpful to decide in advance on a set of positive habits to consciously draw from – both as a baseline from which to operate and as a set of positive behaviours to focus on if and when things get tough on the journey. It might be helpful to think of these habits, or rituals, as your anchors – stopping you from drifting off course and slipping into any bad *old* habits that you are trying to escape from. I have created a list for you of the "anchors" I have found to be the most supportive for me over the years.

I'd suggest doing these things every day if you want to see differences fast (they can, of course, be done in any order that suits you):

- Wake at the same time each day: This is a great way to get your body into a positive, regular rhythm and will help you feel more grounded.

- Make your bed in the morning: This seemingly simple "act of will" can have a huge impact on your self-esteem, and is used by both the SAS and Navy SEALs among other elite forces to teach discipline.

- Gently stretch out each part of your body as soon as you get up in the morning, from your head to your toes – to awaken both body and mind.

- Meditate for at least 12 minutes: Ideally, do this both morning and night, but once is better than nothing! Revisit the Loving Kindness Meditation on page 46 for inspiration.

- Rejuvenate your face: Spend a little time each day doing either the Natural Face-Lift Exercise on page 162, the Lymphatic Drainage Facial on page 165 or the Acupressure Facial Routine on page 168.

- Make a delicious smoothie with green leafy veggies (see also the recipes in Chapter 6, pages 88–9, and at JayneyGoddard.org).

- Brush and floss your teeth: This will help you feel fresher and brighter.

- Schedule in time for exercise: It's wise to vary this from day to day between resistance training, for strength, and more mindful forms of exercise, such as Pilates, yoga, tai chi or qigong, also being sure to fit in aerobic activities, some exercise outside, in nature, if possible and maybe also some exercise with others to factor in some sociability too. (See Chapter 12 for more on this.)

  In Week 1, I suggest avoiding any resistance training given this week is all about "letting go" before you "build up". But, once you move past Week 1, your exercise plan should ideally look something like this, with at least three sessions of aerobic exercise fitted in wherever you can, even if just brisk outdoor walks of 30 minutes or more:

Day 1: Resistance training
Day 2: Mindful exercise
Day 3: Resistance training
Day 4: Mindful exercise
Day 5: Resistance training
Day 6: Mindful exercise
Day 7: Rest

- Drink plenty of water: We are all different when it comes to how much water we need, so it's best to monitor yourself regularly. If your pee is very pale or clear, you're adequately hydrated. If not, get pouring! Please note: tea, coffee and other caffeinated drinks are not hydrating.

- Implement a simple wind-down routine: This might include switching off the TV, your phone and any other screens half an hour or an hour before bed, and then spending time writing in a gratitude journal (see page 55), having a warm bath, doing your facial acupressure (see page 168) or burning some essential oils in a diffuser (see page 199).

- Get good sleep: 7 hours a night is ideal, or maybe a little less or more depending on your individual needs (see pages 213–4 for more on this).

I'd also suggest doing the following activities at least once a week:

- Revisit your list of Mindset Phrases on Day 1 of each week to get you into an optimal, focused, positive frame of mind for the week ahead.

- Do an activity that can be described as "enriching", such as spending time with friends to tap into the revitalizing powers of sociability (see Chapter 16), doing a selfless good deed to tap into the positive power of loving kindness (see page 56) or spending time in nature to tap into its power to simultaneously calm, heal and inspire pure awe. The options here are endless, so be as creative as you like when deciding what to do.

- Practise the deeply relaxing Yoga Nidra technique (see page 216) for 20 minutes either before you go to bed, or once you are in bed and lying down comfortably. It can actually be done at any time, but just before bed is particularly beneficial to help you get a good night's sleep.

WEEK 1
SIMPLIFYING, DETOXING AND DECLUTTERING

The main theme of this, the first week of the Rewind Plan, is to "let go" of anything that is no longer helping you move forward as you wish in life. This decluttering will be a way of creating space for more of the good things you want, sending yourself a strong message that this is a new beginning. Think of it like a deep spring-clean that will leave you refreshed, clearer about your future and feeling equipped to make age-rewind changes to become healthier and more vibrant.

Note: If you smoke, now is the ideal time to stop! Even if you've struggled to do so in the past, do please try again in the spirit of this energy of letting go for a healthier, more vibrant future.

Nutrition and Supplement Support

It's important if you're serious about rewinding your body clock that you take nutritional steps in line with the information shared about a healthy, natural diet in Chapter 6. Understanding the rationale (both scientific and ethical) behind why a plant-based, wholefood diet will help you embark on this path if it's one that feels right for you. As you are cleansing and clearing this week, pay particular attention to incorporating plenty of high-fibre options into your meals.

I also recommend taking supplements to support you in this time of change, such as any of the adaptogenic herbs on pages 122–4. Other especially helpful ones in this detoxifying stage include chlorella, milk thistle and psyllium husk. Just be sure to read the instructions on the packaging and check for allergies and contraindications.

Day 1

- Do all your Daily Rewind Habits.
- Revisit your Mindset Phrases (as discussed on page 226) to set you up positively for the week ahead and, if it feels right, choose one or two of them that feel particularly relevant to this week's theme, and/or create a new Mindset Phrase to rekindle your enthusiasm. What do you want to discard that no longer serves you?
- Set aside time to go through your fridge and food cupboards and get rid of anything that you know is unhealthy after reading this book. In particular, anything that contains any of the following ingredients:
  - Hydrogenated oil
  - Partially hydrogenated oils (also known as trans fats)
  - Foods containing high levels of omega 6 oils (corn oil, cottonseed oil, safflower oil, soybean oil, sunflower oil)
  - Refined sugars (including anything that ends in an "ose" – fructose, glucose, maltose, sucrose, etc., or containing sugar alcohols that end in "ol" – sorbitol, maltitol, etc.)
  - High-salt foods, mixes and seasonings
- If you are keen to follow a plant-based, wholefood diet or become vegan, today is also the day to get rid of any meat, fish, eggs and dairy.
- Either remove all sources of caffeine, or hide them so that they're not in temptation's way. If you're a light caffeine user, you might choose to cut out caffeine straightaway. If you're a heavy user, it's better to reduce exposure gradually over the week, as you may get withdrawal symptoms, such as headaches. These won't be severe but may be nagging. If this does happen, just drink lots of water and take extra vitamin C or eat more fruit. Any time you feel like a coffee or tea, make yourself a herbal tea instead; dandelion, fennel or milk thistle would be particularly good choices to aid with this week's cleansing.
- Rearrange whatever is left in your fridge and food cupboards so that it is clean, neat and organized, and check any remaining use-by dates.
- Do approximately an hour of mindful exercise, such as yoga, Pilates, tai chi or qi gong.
- If you have time, fit in a brisk walk, even if this is only to the shops and back, or a quick circuit of the local park.
- Practise pre-bed Yoga Nidra (see page 216), using this as your intention: "I consciously cleanse myself, and my environment, of anything that I no longer need, or that is holding me back in any way – making space for health, freedom, lightness, energy, happiness and youthful vibrancy."

Day 2

- Do all your Daily Rewind Habits.
- Go shopping for healthy food based on what you learnt in Chapter 6. Feel free to look up recipes on my website, JayneyGoddard.org, to get you started. Top tip: Don't go shopping when hungry!
- Buy some Epsom salts in readiness for starting your resistance training next week (to build strength and stamina). This way, you'll be able to take restorative baths, which you'll be glad of!
- Invest in an organic cleanser or make-up remover for yourself, and if you use cotton balls or pads, ensure that these are organic too.
- Take part in an "enrichment" activity of your choice that both makes you feel good and has far-reaching wellness benefits, whether going for a walk in the great outdoors, attending a dance class, going to an art gallery with friends, watching the night sky, or anything else that appeals.

Day 3

- Do all your Daily Rewind Habits.
- Go for a brisk walk outside, preferably for at least 30 minutes.
- Today is the day to declutter any toxic cleaning products from your home, using the information on pages 179/201 as a starting point.
- Check the labels of your shampoos, shower gels, cosmetics etc. for harmful chemicals such as the hormone disruptors mentioned on page 178. Ideally, replace them with organic products that are free from nasties.
- Do some mindful exercise, such as yoga, tai chi, Pilates or mindful walking; the duration is up to you.

Day 4

- Do all your Daily Rewind Habits.
- Gather together some nutritious, plant-based recipes that you would like to try – to replace any "bad habit" meals that you sometimes (or maybe often) have, such as pre-packaged "ready meals" or takeaways.
- Shake things up by doing something that you've never done before: go to an event, try a new sport or class, go for a walk in a new neighbourhood – whatever takes your fancy.
- Take part in an "enrichment" activity of your choice.

Day 5

- Do all your Daily Rewind Habits.
- Go for a brisk walk outside, preferably for at least 30 minutes.
- Take a look through your wardrobe and/or drawers. Are there any clothes that you haven't worn in a while, that you no longer like or that no longer fit you? Can you give any of these to friends or donate them to charity? Take this time to really pare things back, keeping only what makes you feel great about yourself. If you have a lot of clothes, you might need to spread this out over several days.
- Do some mindful exercise of your choice.

Day 6

- Do all your Daily Rewind Habits.
- Take an inventory of the main people in your life. Could you class any of them as "frenemies"? (See page 190 for more on this.) If so, consider how you might reduce or even eliminate contact with them. And if not, might there be creative ways of *managing* your contact with them?
- If you feel comfortable doing so, make today a juice-feasting day. Ideally, make your own juice – see my recipes on page 87. You'll need about 1.7l (3.5 pints) of juice to last you through the day. I prefer to make my juice fresh each time if at all possible.
- Do some mindful exercise of your choice.

Day 7

- Do all your Daily Rewind Habits.
- Take a break from all forms of technology and media: TV, your mobile phone, the internet, newspapers etc. How does this feel? Most people find it incredibly liberating to take time away from screens and not to be constantly bombarded with news for a change. Is this something that you might want to continue one day a week even beyond the 3-week plan?
- Also make today a day of non-judgement, allowing any propensity toward judging yourself and others to fall away. Step outside of yourself, simply observe things as they happen and let them float by.
- Take part in an "enrichment" activity of your choice.

WEEK 2

BUILDING UP, GROWING AND EXPANDING

Now that you've made room for more wonderful, life-enhancing goodness in your life by letting go in Week 1 of many of the things that no longer serve you – from harmful chemicals in the home, unhealthy foods and unwanted clothes to negative thoughts and negative people – it's time to spend the next seven days focusing on what new positive qualities you want to bring *into* your life: foods, drink, thoughts, habits, activities, people and all the rest. What will make you feel most youthful, dynamic, happy and vibrant, and therefore bring you the wellness benefits that will start to rewind your body clock?

Nutrition and Supplement Support

I hope you're not finding it too tough to incorporate the health-enhancing nutritional choices discussed in Chapter 6 into your diet, whether you've gone fully plant-based or not. Might you even be starting to enjoy it? I do hope so. Remember that there is plenty of recipe inspiration for you on my website should you need it. This week, given that the focus is on building and strengthening, I'd like you to particularly ensure that you're getting adequate levels of all macronutrients, including protein.

If, during Week 1, you decided to supplement your diet with any of the adaptogens from pages 122–3, then it's sensible to continue to do so this week, too, as this will help provide you with the balance and stamina that you'll need for both this week and next. Just remember that it's best when taking herbs to take one week off in any month, so that your body doesn't build up a tolerance to them.

Day 1

- Do all your Daily Rewind Habits.
- Revisit your Mindset Phrases (as discussed on page 226) to set you up positively for the week ahead and, if it feels right, choose one or two of them that feel particularly relevant to this week's theme, and/or create a new Mindset Phrase to rekindle your enthusiasm. What are you gaining from embarking on the Rewind Journey?
- Go for a brisk walk outside, preferably for at least 30 minutes.
- Reach out to an old friend who you haven't seen in a long time, such as someone from school. We all have those good old friends that we occasionally lose contact with. If you connect with them, you're likely to benefit greatly from chatting about the past. This is a partial "immersion" process (as outlined on page 11) that will help to rewind your body clock by bringing all those things from your youth to mind.
- Start resistance training today; I suggest hiring a personal trainer at the start if you're not used to working with weights. Remember to alternate days between this and mindful activities, as per the guidance on page 228.
- Take a warm, relaxing bath with Epsom salts to relieve any muscle soreness from your training.
- Practise pre-bed Yoga Nidra (see page 216), using this as your intention: "I am consciously bringing thoughts and processes into my life that build a firm foundation of wellbeing, in body, mind and spirit. By nurturing my development in this way, I ensure success in achieving my wellness goals."

Day 2

- Do all your Daily Rewind Habits.
- Stock up on healthy foods, based on my guidance in Chapter 6, as well as on your own additional research if desired, of course.
- Listen to some music from the past that really makes you feel happy – and dance around your living room to it like no one's watching! This is another "immersion" Rewind practice, as mentioned above.
- Visit or go out with family or friends. Also consider what you can do to create new friendships and increase your social support network.
- Do some mindful exercise of your choice.
- Take part in an "enrichment" activity of your choice.

Day 3

- Do all your Daily Rewind Habits.
- Go for a brisk walk outside, preferably for at least 30 minutes.
- Make contact with an elderly person who you've not managed to keep in touch with over the years and rekindle that relationship. Or reach out to a local elderly person in your area who maybe lives alone and could do with occasional company. This will have a double-whammy age-rewind effect as it taps into both the anti-ageing benefits of sociability (see page 185) and kindness and compassion (see page 186).
- Do your resistance training.
- Take part in an "enrichment" activity of your choice.

Day 4

- Do all your Daily Rewind Habits.
- Research local groups in leisure areas that interest you, whether that be theatre, dance, swimming, knitting, chess or whatever else. And choose one to get involved with so that you can reap the benefits of not just the social side of things (see Chapter 16) but also the cognitive skills involved, whether remembering lines or dance steps, having to be spatially aware in the pool, the hand-eye coordination involved in craft activities or the strategic thinking involved in a game like chess.
- Build your confidence by doing something completely outside your comfort zone, whether performing at karaoke, reciting a poem in public or signing up for a long trek! Taking action like this creates "eustress" – the good form of stress that gives us a shot of enlivening adrenaline and other stress hormones but doesn't produce a damaging, long-term (chronic) upsurge in cortisol.
- Do some mindful exercise of your choice.

Day 5

- Do all your Daily Rewind Habits.
- Go for a brisk walk outside, preferably for at least 30 minutes.
- Do your resistance training.
- Harness the power of music to boost your workout today by choosing a playlist that you not only love but that has a nice fast tempo, as we tend

to subconsciously alter the pace of our steps or movements to stay in time with the beat of the music. Faster-paced music has been shown to make working out more enjoyable, too. It doesn't matter which genre of music you like – anything is fine – as long as it has some pace.

Day 6

- Do all your Daily Rewind Habits.
- Do some brain-trainers, such as crosswords, Sudoku, or online brain-training exercises. It doesn't matter what it is, as long as it's something that you'll enjoy and that will also challenge you.
- Do some mindful exercise of your choice.
- Take part in an "enrichment" activity of your choice.

Day 7

Today is all about rest and contemplation, so we will repeat certain elements from Week 1:

- Do all your Daily Rewind Habits.
- As on Day 7, Week 1: Take a break from all technology and media.
- Also as on Day 7, Week 1: Make today a day of non-judgement, allowing any propensity toward judging yourself and others fall away. Step outside of yourself and simply observe things as they happen.
- Do a random act of kindness (see page 188) – no matter how big or small, whether for someone you know or for a stranger. Consider getting your friends and family involved in this too; doing something like this together can be particularly bonding. How can you and your loved ones make a difference in someone's day today? Be a kindness ninja and see just how good it makes you, in turn, feel.

WEEK 3

CONSOLIDATING, STRENGTHENING AND SUSTAINING

The focus this week is on consolidating and locking in your new-found positive habits and behaviours so that you can sustain them – and hopefully build on them, moving forward. After all, this 21-day plan is only meant to be the *start* of your Rewind Journey, so it's important that it really makes some fundamental differences to how you think, to how you approach things, to how you structure and fill your days and weeks – and, most importantly, to how you feel about yourself, as mindset is key!

Nutrition and Supplement Support

Continue to eat as healthily as you can and take your choice of supplements from Weeks 1 and 2, remembering that you'll need to take a break from the herbs in particular next week as the rule for herbs is "three weeks on, one week off", unless advised to the contrary by a professional herbalist.

Day 1

- Do all your Daily Rewind Habits.
- Revisit your Mindset Phrases (as discussed on page 226) to set you up positively for the week ahead and, if it feels right, choose one or two of them that feel particularly relevant to this week's theme, and/or create a new Mindset Phrase to rekindle your enthusiasm. What lies at the core of how you want to nurture yourself and live life moving forward?

- Set aside a little time to take stock of how everything you've been doing for the past two weeks has been focused on building a platform from which to move forward into a happier, healthier future. You may want to use positive visualization (see page 61) to envisage how you will *feel* in this future.
- Do your resistance training.
- Take part in an "enrichment" activity of your choice.
- Practise pre-bed Yoga Nidra (see page 216), using this as your intention: "My focus this week is to sustain life-affirming habits so that I can take these forward into a happy, healthy, ageless future. I now know what I have to do to lead a happy, healthy life and to rewind my body clock."

Day 2

- Do all your Daily Rewind Habits.
- Go for a brisk walk outside, preferably for at least 30 minutes.
- Set aside a little dedicated time to think about, and write down, a range of active ways in which you will sustain your new healthy habits moving forward, whether from within this plan, elsewhere in the book or beyond.
- Invite friends round, ask them to bring music they loved when they were a teenager and reset your physiology to a much younger age by dancing the night away together – maybe even having a slumber party!
- Do some mindful exercise of your choice.

Day 3

- Do all your Daily Rewind Habits.
- Make a list of comedies you love and watch one of them today; laughter really is the best medicine. George Bernard Shaw wrote, "You don't stop laughing when you grow old, you grow old when you stop laughing."
- Do your resistance training.
- Take part in an "enrichment" activity of your choice.

Day 4

- Do all your Daily Rewind Habits.
- Go for a brisk walk outside, preferably for at least 30 minutes.
- Sign up for an extreme challenge of some kind that allows you to take

advantage of the anti-ageing effects of "eustress" even more than you did in Week 2. Maybe something like parachuting, taking a flying lesson or handling a snake? A challenge is a personal thing, so dig deep, figure out what will get your heart racing – and do it!

- If you find a challenging activity you enjoy – provided you are dealing with stress well and feeling quite resilient – there's no reason you shouldn't make these adrenaline-shot activities more regular. In this way, you'll strengthen your ability to deal with stressors that life throws up at random.
- Do some mindful exercise of your choice.

Day 5

- Do all your Daily Rewind Habits.
- Give someone a gift. This doesn't have to be anything big, but the more meaningful and connected to the recipient it is, the better. Maybe make something – a cake, a piece of art, a haiku or a handmade card. Acts of kindness and generosity are one of the most potent Rewind strategies available to us (see page 188 for more on this).
- Take a moment to think creatively about ways in which you can lock in this generosity habit and make it more sustainable, whether selecting certain days to perform random acts of kindness, sharing regular time with people who will benefit from your company, or whatever else.
- Do your resistance training.
- Take part in an "enrichment" activity of your choice.

Day 6

- Do all your Daily Rewind Habits.
- Go for a brisk walk outside, preferably for at least 30 minutes.
- Set aside a little time to think about someone who has wronged you and try to find a place in your heart from which to forgive them. Use the Metta (Loving Kindness) Meditation on page 56 to help you with this by developing compassion toward the person. When we hold onto a grudge it restricts how happy we can truly be, whereas when we make a conscious decision to forgive, we free ourselves to soar.
- Do some mindful exercise of your choice.

Day 7

Today is all about rest and contemplation, so we will repeat certain elements from both Week 1 and Week 2:

- Do all your Daily Rewind Habits.
- As on Day 7, Weeks 1 and 2: Take a break from all media and technology. Might you be able to get your friends involved too this time?
- As on Day 7, Weeks 1 and 2: Make today a day of non-judgement and gentleness towards both yourself and others.
- As on Day 7, Week 2: Plan random acts of kindness. As with last week, get friends and family in on the act!

Next Steps on Your Rewind Journey

Congratulations! You've reached the end of your 21-Day Rewind Plan. By doing all the activities that it entails you have rewired your brain to choose things that will start you on the path to being happier and more resilient to stress, as well as fitter and leaner, with more stamina.

I recommend that you continue with your new daily habits after the 21 days as these are the absolute cornerstone of the programme; that you add some of the other suggestions from the plan into your days; and that you also add other preferred activities from throughout the rest of the book – in order to tailor your routine to your *individual* needs and desires.

For example, you might add the lemon drink from page 72 to your morning ritual, make a few of the "Luscious Locks" treatments from Chapter 14 daily habits, make a soothing exercise such as the Relaxation Response (see page 62) or Taoist Longevity Breathing (see pages 130–31) a regular event, or any other combination that feels helpful and relevant to you.

The number of activities you add will, of course, depend on how much time you have to dedicate to the Rewind cause each day and week – and also on how well you plan your time at the start of each week. I highly recommend that you use a journal to mark out exactly when you intend to do what each day in advance – in order to stay feeling on top of things.

It's also good to look back at both your "Motivations and Goals" and your present-tense "Mindset Phrases" regularly, and change anything that strikes you. The more you do this, the more engrained your new positive habits will become – and the easier the Rewind Journey will feel. Remember: YOU are in the driving seat – and YOU are in control of your future health, happiness and health-span. You have way more control over how you age – and now you have all the tools you need to get going.

CONCLUSION
WHERE TO GO FROM HERE

It can help immensely to have companions alongside you for support and motivation, so why not get some friends involved with your age-rewind adventure too? People power! I have set up a private Facebook group so that you can share your age-rewind journey with other people who are going through the steps that you are. It can really help to motivate you if you have a group of like-minded supporters. It is called "Rewind Your Body Clock with Jayney Goddard" and I'm in the group too, so you'll have direct access to me if you have any questions or need any support at all along the way. This will allow you to use the power of sociability and accountability to support you in your journey.

Whatever the next steps are that you choose to take on this exciting journey, remember that it is never too late to begin, no matter your age or state of health. I have people in my programmes and who come to see me in my clinic and attend my retreats who are healthy and fit – and want to stay that way – right through to people who are dealing with chronic degenerative disease – who know that there are solutions and that lifestyle is the biggest part of the battle. Wherever you are on your journey, remember that you are not alone. Reading this book is just the beginning, and together we can rewind your body clock.

Remember, you have so much more control than you probably ever realized before, so let's go for it with a fresh positivity, knowing that all the recommendations in this book are supported by strong scientific research – even though they are "natural" in origin.

The trick to success with your biological age-reversal journey is to begin to make the changes *now*, because, if you don't, you'll lose momentum and find yourself in the exact same position in a month, a year, or more.

The sooner you get going, the sooner you will see results. So keep me posted with your progress. I'm excited to hear how you get on! Meanwhile, I wish you youthful vitality, health and happiness.

With love,
Jayney

USEFUL RESOURCES

All of the practices, tests and remedies that I recommend in this book rely on my extensive academic research and studies. However, I also know that your time is precious, which is why I have avoided adding a lengthy reference section to this book. If, however, you'd like to read any of the research or studies for yourself, you'll find a full list of detailed references for all the relevant publications, including research papers, on my website, JayneyGoddard.org

That said, there are a number of resources that I have chosen for you and included below, as I consider them to be truly "stand-out" in the field of happiness, wellness and youthfulness. In science, we all stand on the shoulders of giants, and these authors, organizations and film-makers are indeed giants in the natural youth arena. Some of them I know personally, and some I've yet to meet, but all of these talented people are making huge contributions to society and to the planet, with their brilliant insight and wisdom, so I recommend that you make the following resources a vital part of your Rewind Journey.

Recommended Books

Dr Elizabeth Blackburn and Dr Elissa Epel, *The Telomere Effect: A Revolutionary Approach to Living Younger, Healthier, Longer* (2018)

Brendan Brazier and Hugh Jackman, *Thrive: The Vegan Nutrition Guide to Optimal Performance in Sports and Life: The Whole Food Way to Lose Weight, Reduce Stress, and Stay Healthy for Life* (2008)

Dr T Colin Campbell, *Whole: Rethinking the Science of Nutrition* (2014)

Robert Cheeke and Vanessa Espinosa, *Plant Based Muscle* (2017)

Dr Sara Gottfried, MD, *Younger: A Breakthrough Program to Reset Your Genes, Reverse Aging, and Turn Back the Clock 10 Years* (2018)

Dr Michael Greger and Gene Stone, *How Not To Die: Discover the Foods Scientifically Proven to Prevent and Reverse Disease* (2017)

David R. Hamilton, PhD, *The Five Side Effects of Kindness* (2017)

Matthieu Ricard, *Happiness: A Guide to Developing Life's Most Important Skill*, Kindle Edition (2015)

Useful Websites

JayneyGoddard.org This is my own website, which is an incredibly useful additional resource for everything discussed in this book. It includes information, recipes and so much more that will enhance your life in myriad ways and support you on your journey to "Rewind Your Body Clock". Plus, this is where to log in if you want to store and track your age-rewind test results from the Self-Assessment (pages 19–22) securely, online.

"Jayney Goddard" YouTube channel Here you'll find a wide range of videos on all sorts of "Rewind" topics, right across the board. I love that it allows me to interact with you directly and answer any questions you may have. Also – if you subscribe to the channel and hit the little "bell" icon you'll be notified each time I upload a new video, so you'll never miss out. See also my Instagram page, "JayneyGoddard", for similar material.

The-CMA.org.uk The Complementary Medical Association (CMA) is the world's largest and most respected professional membership association for complementary and integrative medical practitioners, students, training schools/colleges, retreats and spas. The site has an astounding 7,500+ articles on every aspect of natural healthcare that you can imagine, and a free-to-use database to find a practitioner near you – or a training school, if you are looking at becoming qualified in a natural health discipline.

BSLM.com The British Society of Lifestyle Medicine website contains an abundance of useful information and also offers professional training in becoming a fully qualified Lifestyle Medicine Consultant, with new courses emerging all the time. Well worth checking out, particularly if you are considering a career transition – perhaps inspired by this book.

DrFrankSabatino.com This is an excellent site full of information on every aspect of living a healthy lifestyle and eating a plant-based, wholefood diet in the "real world". Acknowledged as one of the world's leading experts in water-only fasting, Dr Sabatino also provides invaluable information on this.

PCRM.org On this website for the Physician's Committee for Responsible Medicine you'll find everything you need to know about plant-based, wholefood eating – including robust scientific research about transitioning to a healthy, plant-based diet – and lots of recipes and encouragement.

Suggested Films

Cowspiracy Follow the shocking, yet humorous, adventures of an aspiring environmentalist as he courageously seeks to find the solution to the most pressing environmental issues and a true path to sustainability.

Earthlings A chronicle of the day-to-day practices of the largest industries in the world, all of which rely on animals for profit, using hidden cameras and never-before-seen footage. Graphic in parts but important viewing.

Fat, Sick and Nearly Dead An inspirational film – ideal for anyone who doubts that lifestyle changes can make a difference. Overweight by 100lbs, loaded up on cortico-steroids and suffering from a debilitating autoimmune disease, Joe Cross has lost hope of ever getting well. Watch his progress as he embarks on an incredible juicing adventure. Wonderful!

Forks Over Knives This film examines the claim that most, if not all, of the degenerative diseases that we associate with poor ageing can be controlled by rejecting our present menu of animal-based, processed foods.

Live and Let Live This feature documentary examines our relationship with animals, the history of veganism and the ethical, environmental and health reasons that move people to go vegan.

Simply Raw: Reversing Diabetes in 30 Days This film follows diabetes patients on a quest to overcome the disease by going on a raw vegan diet.

Supersize Me Documentary-maker Morgan Spurlock embarks on an "adventure" in which he eats only "supersized" junk food. Medics track his progress over the experiment and the results are truly shocking.

Vegucated This is a guerrilla-style documentary that follows three meat- and cheese-loving New Yorkers who reluctantly agree to adopt a vegan diet for six weeks and learn what it's all about. It's a real eye-opener.

ABOUT THE AUTHOR

Jayney Goddard is one of the world's leading experts in the fields of complementary medicine and natural health. She is a broadcaster, author, lecturer and journalist and an acknowledged thought leader in the health care arena. Initially a ballerina, Jayney "accidentally" joined the circus as an aerial artiste, which required travel to some of the most far-flung and primitive places in the world. During this time, when there was no access to conventional medicines, she witnessed first-hand the phenomenal power of natural, folk medicines. And it was this that inspired her to train in a range of complementary medical disciplines.

Jayney is now founder and president of The Complementary Medicine Association (The CMA) and founder and co-chair of the British Society of Lifestyle Medicine. She has a Master of Science post-graduate degree from UCLan, England; trained in Mind/Body Medicine at Harvard Medical School, USA, under Dr Herbert Benson (the "father" of Mind/Body Medicine); and runs an international practice in which she uses a range of natural medicine approaches to help clients reach their fullest health potential. Due to Jayney's extensive training, she always ensures her recommendations are grounded in robust scientific research – so that both her clients, and readers, know her suggestions are fully proven to work.

Jayney is passionate about working with people suffering from chronic lifestyle-related conditions, as she herself experienced a life-threatening illness that left her wheelchair-bound for ten years. At her lowest point, she was in hospice care, weighing only 5.5 stone (35kg; 77lbs), and not expected to survive. As a result, she aged dramatically from a "biological" perspective, measuring in at 55 when she was, in reality, only 36. However, Jayney knew in her heart that she had the ability to beat the illness via natural methods, and she did! After coming up with all the recommendations that she now writes about in this book, Jayney managed not only to get healthy – but also to rewind her own body clock in the process! Now 55, Jayney's biological clock shows that her body, mind and physical capabilities are a mere 27! She says, "Mindset is 99 per cent of the battle. If I can do it, you can too! And I'm here to be your guide on this incredible journey."

To find out more about Jayney and her work, go to JayneyGoddard.org.

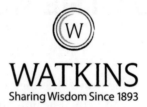

WATKINS

Sharing Wisdom Since 1893

The story of Watkins began in 1893, when scholar of esotericism John Watkins founded our bookshop, inspired by the lament of his friend and teacher Madame Blavatsky that there was nowhere in London to buy books on mysticism, occultism or metaphysics. That moment marked the birth of Watkins, soon to become the publisher of many of the leading lights of spiritual literature, including Carl Jung, Rudolf Steiner, Alice Bailey and Chögyam Trungpa.

Today, the passion at Watkins Publishing for vigorous questioning is still resolute. Our stimulating and groundbreaking list ranges from ancient traditions and complementary medicine to the latest ideas about personal development, holistic wellbeing and consciousness exploration. We remain at the cutting edge, committed to publishing books that change lives.

DISCOVER MORE AT:

www.watkinspublishing.com

Read our blog

Watch and listen to
our authors in action

Sign up to
our mailing list

We celebrate conscious, passionate, wise and happy living.

Be part of that community by visiting

f /watkinspublishing   **🐦** @watkinswisdom

▶ /watkinsbooks   **📷** @watkinswisdom